"Dr. Melvin Kaplan's fascinating book provides vivid accounts of his important work with dozens of patients he has treated, using yoked prism glasses to increase their awareness of our wide spatial environment. Dr. Kaplan's terrific writing should encourage research into the benefits of vision therapy that will convince the medical community of the effectiveness of his approach."

—*Albert Yonas, Professor of Child Psychology, Institute of Child Development, University of Minnesota*

"In these pages, Dr. Kaplan presents a novel interactive approach to addressing severe visual deficits. Through compelling patient stories, he shows that symptoms ranging from anxiety and learning disabilities to toe-walking and scoliosis are not 'problems' but rather the solutions patients create to compensate for visual dysfunction. Dr. Kaplan shows how these symptoms can guide clinicians to correct visual problems and, as a result, change lives for the better."

—*Dr. Ned Hallowell, Founder of The Hallowell Center for Cognitive and Emotional Health, New York and Boston*

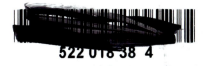

by the same author

Seeing Through New Eyes
Changing the Lives of Children with Autism, Asperger Syndrome
and other Developmental Disabilities Through Vision Therapy
Melvin Kaplan
Foreword by Stephen Edelson
ISBN 978 1 84310 800 9
eISBN 978 1 84642 247 8

THE SECRETS
IN THEIR
Eyes

Transforming the Lives
of People with Cognitive,
Emotional, Learning, or
Movement Disorders or
Autism by Changing the
Visual Software of the Brain

MELVIN KAPLAN

FOREWORD BY MANUEL CASANOVA

Jessica Kingsley *Publishers*
London and Philadelphia

First published in 2015
by Jessica Kingsley Publishers
73 Collier Street
London N1 9BE, UK
and
400 Market Street, Suite 400
Philadelphia, PA 19106, USA

www.jkp.com

Library of Congress Cataloging in Publication Data
Kaplan, Melvin, 1929- , author.
  The secrets in their eyes : transforming the lives of
people with cognitive, emotional, learning or
movement disorders or autism by changing the visual
software of the brain / Melvin Kaplan.
       p. ; cm.
  ISBN 978-1-84905-736-3 (alk. paper)
  I. Title.
  [DNLM: 1. Vision Disorders--complications--Case Reports.
2. Vision Disorders--therapy--Case Reports.
3. Developmental Disabilities--etiology--Case Reports.
4. Mental Disorders--etiology--Case Reports. 5.
Neurobehavioral Manifestations--Case Reports. WW 140]
  RE725
  617.7--dc23
                              2014044138

British Library Cataloguing in Publication Data
A CIP catalogue record for this book is available from the British Library

ISBN 978 1 84905 736 3
eISBN 978 1 78450 140 2

Printed and bound in Great Britain

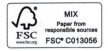

To my wife Ellen, my children Marc,
Stuart, David and the memory of Jeffrey

Contents

Section 4 Conclusion

FOREWORD

"He's lost his sense of space," said Mel, examining a child in my clinic. Then he grabbed a small beanie bag and placed it on top of the child's head. "The weight will serve to center him," Mel added. In less than a minute the tantrum faded away.

This was one of my many experiences with Melvin Kaplan as he examined patients with autism spectrum disorders in my laboratory, where we were recruiting volunteers for a prism study.

I'd first met Melvin Kaplan several years ago through an introduction by a mutual friend, Steve Edelson, the Executive Director for the Autism Research Institute (ARI). It was Steve who arranged to have us work together on the prism study. I happen to do research involving autism, and Mel happens to be one of the pioneering figures in the field of Behavioral Optometry and visual rehabilitation. Putting us together seemed to be a perfect fit.

To be truthful, I'd never heard of Behavioral Optometry before meeting Mel. As I caught up on the subject, I learned that there are only a few health-related professionals in this field. Behavioral Optometry is derived from an amalgam of ophthalmology, psychology, and education. It obviously helps going into the field if, like Mel, you are a little bit of a bookworm, you're intelligent, and you have assorted interests.

Mel's "talking approach" was quite evident at the clinic. In dealing with children and their parents, Mel was careful to explain his findings and thought processes in layman's terms.

This allowed me to learn a lot from Mel's commonsensical approach to neurodevelopmental conditions.

In many neurodevelopmental conditions, individuals lack spatial awareness and have trouble with coordination, which consequently manifests as challenging behaviors.

With the aid of Mel's techniques, patients exhibit significant improvements. Sometimes, these are obvious at the very first meeting. Other times, patients exhibit progress over many months while undergoing therapy. Indeed, it sometimes takes time for the brain to rewire itself—that is, to change the basic blueprint of brain connectivity. We have used Mel's technique as a complementary approach to our own therapeutic endeavors, and Mel's clinical acumen has inspired me to become a better physician. Let Mel talk to you, tell you his story, and describe what he has learned from his patients. Whether you are a professional, a parent, or a person dealing with a neurodevelopmental condition yourself, it may well change your life.

Manuel F. Casanova M.D.
Gottfried and Gisela Kolb Endowed Chair in Psychiatry
Professor of Psychiatry, Neurology, Anatomy and
Bioengineering
Vice Chairman of Psychiatry
University of Louisville

OVERVIEW

The fastest way to change behavior is through a lens.

VISION THERAPY PIONEER A.M. SKEFFINGTON

1

VISUAL PERCEPTUAL PROBLEMS

An Introduction

When our visual system is working correctly, it provides us with more information in less time than any other sense. Scientists estimate that 80 percent of our impressions come through our eyes, and it's these impressions that largely determine who we are and who we can become. Biology gives each of us a brain; but our vision, more than any other sense, determines the way we function in the world.

Sighted people can only reach their full potential, however, when their vision is accurate. In short, stable vision is necessary for achieving a stable perception of our world. If deficits in the visual processing software of the brain stop us from developing a stable gaze, we may "see" in the traditional sense—but we will not perceive our world correctly, because we can't receive, integrate, decode, and interpret information about where objects are. In fact, we may not even perceive *ourselves* correctly.

Many of my patients have normal or near-normal focal (central) vision, which allows them to identify objects. But they have unstable ambient (peripheral) vision. Ambient vision constantly informs us about our changing world—telling us where we are in space, and where objects in our environment are—and when the brain software involved in ambient vision is faulty, we "mis-see" our world and our place in it.

If you suffer from a visual perceptual problem, you know that such "mis-seeing" can be life-altering. For instance, reading may be stressful or even painful, making schoolwork impossible. Driving may be terrifying. Objects may seem to rush at you suddenly, or to disappear for no reason. You may have tunnel vision that effectively makes you blind to much of your world. You may feel clumsy or awkward around other people. You may even see the patterns on your wallpaper moving, or feel as if the walls of your house are closing in on you. Your symptoms may be severe enough for you to receive a diagnosis of anxiety, depression, learning disability, schizophrenia, or even autism.

If you are experiencing visual symptoms like these, you may feel frustrated, depressed, anxious, or even terrified—especially if doctor after doctor fails to help you. But the exciting news is that the proper vision therapy techniques can correct these problems, no matter how old you are or how severe your symptoms are.

In fact, as you will see, the symptoms you're experiencing are the very key to overcoming your problems. In this book, I'll explain why these symptoms are actually solutions—your brain's way of compensating for inaccurate visual information—and why they can point to interventions that can ameliorate your visual deficits permanently. Over the decades, I've successfully treated thousands of patients from all over the world simply by letting these patients' symptoms steer me to the correct interventions.

These interventions involve a powerful tool called "ambient yoked prisms." By transforming light, yoked prisms alter visual stimulation from the environment, in turn transforming perception and cognition. This can lead to dramatic improvements in attention as well as reductions in visual stress.

To show you how powerful these transformations can be, I'd like to introduce you to three patients whose lives were changed by visual management programs.

Peter's story

Peter was 19 when he first came to see me. He was one of the smartest young men I'd ever met—in fact, his IQ was off the charts—but he'd dropped out of college in his first semester. Now he was losing job after job, and his future was looking dark.

"I can't focus at work," he told me. "I can't organize my thinking. I screw up everything."

Peter's parents initially made appointments for him to see psychiatrists because he was depressed. These doctors gave him many labels: learning disability, poor self-image, attention deficit disorder. One thing they all agreed on was a treatment plan involving medication. But the first medication didn't work. Neither did the next one, or the next one. And as Peter continued to spiral into deeper depression, his parents grew more and more worried.

Looking for real solutions, Peter and his family eventually heard about vision therapy and made an appointment to see me. When I evaluated Peter, I uncovered the reason for his problems: he had severe perceptual visual dysfunction. And I also knew the answer to his problems: a visual management program to retrain his brain to process information more efficiently.

While Peter's eye doctors had given him glasses for his near-sightedness, they'd only looked at the hardware of his eyes—not at the software of his brain, where visual perception occurs. A hardware examination is a conventional test that looks at eye health and refractive issues such as myopia (near-sightedness), hyperopia (far-sightedness), astigmatism (a focusing problem caused by an asymmetrical cornea or lens), and eye alignment. In essence, this exam looks at what's going on in front of the retina. In a software examination, however, I look at what's happening *beyond* the retina. This exam tells me how well a person's brain perceives and processes information in time and space.

My examination of Peter indicated that his myopia was functional, not structural, in nature. This is a common occurrence, often starting when a child reaches the teenage years and educational demands evolve from "learning to read" to the more visually demanding task of "reading to learn." Peter overcompensated for his visual deficits by compressing his visual field to what he could control. As a result, he was unable to quickly gain accurate information about his world.

We scheduled weekly therapy sessions for Peter, starting with disruptive procedures (involving high-magnitude prism lenses, which I describe in Chapter 2) designed to precipitate rapid changes in his perception of both "self" and the outside world. The results were quick and dramatic.

In his sessions, Peter sometimes laughed out loud, overcome with excitement when he saw improvements in his visual skills and felt the changes internally. He'd discovered one of the main principles of therapy: *what you see influences how you feel.*

Within our first five sessions of therapy, Peter returned to school for a course or two. By our tenth session, he'd picked up not just one, but two part-time jobs. By our fifteenth session, he was taking a full load of courses. And by our twenty-fifth session, toward the end of his therapy, he returned to our office with news that had him smiling from ear to ear: he'd made the Dean's List—a list of students achieving the highest academic success.

Peter's remarkable turnaround during his vision therapy occurred not because I changed his eyes (which weren't the source of his problem) but because I changed the way in which his brain perceived his own body and his surroundings. By giving him the tools to correct his visual perceptual impairment, I enabled him to fully see and understand his world—to merge mind, body, and world together into a coherent whole.

Ned's story

Ned, a 27-year-old graduate student, spent much of his first visit telling me about a bizarre ritual he performed. Every day, he would do dozens of one-arm push-ups in an intentional effort to inflict pain on himself. When he reached the point where he could do 25 one-arm push-ups without stress, he started balancing a book—and then several books—on his shoulder to make the exercise more painful.

I asked Ned why he tortured himself in this way. He said he felt that if he could train himself to endure pain, he could cope with the physical pain he felt in his eyes when he read for long periods of time. But his attempted solution failed, and his physical pain led to emotional collapse and admissions to mental hospitals. Fortunately, a psychiatrist with whom I had a long-term professional relationship met Ned and referred him to me.

To people who haven't experienced chronic, severe visual perceptual impairment, Ned's emotional breakdown may sound extreme. But it is difficult to overstate the stress that people like Ned experience as they struggle every day to do things that should be simple but instead are nearly impossible.

Ned had been to other eye doctors in a search for a solution to his eye pain. However, they merely performed standard tests to check the hardware of his eyes. Those exams showed a low degree of myopia, and Ned received glasses to correct his sight to 20/20.

My own hardware exam confirmed Ned's myopia, but that didn't tell me what I needed to know. I got my real clues from my software exam.

This exam revealed that Ned's eyes didn't move efficiently, so he couldn't adjust to changes in his environment quickly enough. He needed to make excessive eye movements and use a great deal of mental energy to find his place while reading, leaving little time for comprehension.

In short, Ned didn't have a problem identifying *what* he saw. Instead, he had a problem finding *where* objects were in his world. This severely affected his ability to perceive his environment in a stable way, leading to impaired performance.

Once I knew what was wrong with Ned, I moved on to the next questions: How, and to what extent, could I change Ned's adaptive behavior?

Based on my clinical findings, I focused in on Ned's issues with sensory memory. Sensory memory is the brain's ability to hold information long enough for it to be transferred to short-term memory.

When Ned read a page, his inefficient eye movements made it impossible for him to stabilize the images of the print on his retina for a sufficient period of time. The transformation of visual sensory input to iconic memory (the formation of a memory of a visual stimulus after viewing it) requires a person to capture the information in less than a second (as compared to auditory processing, which has a three-to-four-second window). In Ned's case, his capacity to transfer visual information into short-term memory came up short. In order for Ned to meet the demands of his courses at school, we needed to address this problem.

I centered Ned's therapy on the goal of improving his gaze control, which would enlarge his sensory gathering field and allow him to capture information more quickly. Once he was able to do this, his sensory memory improved significantly—and his eye pain disappeared.

One day, a reporter from a Toronto paper came to observe our center, and she asked if she could interview one of my patients. Ned was finishing a session and I asked if he would talk to her.

She asked Ned, "How do you experience things now compared to before you started the program here?" And he replied, "Before, when I would be outside I would see a headlight, a tire, and a doorknob and assume it was a car. Now I see the car."

. . . .

How the brain "sees"

Visual information follows two pathways in the brain. One path—the dorsal path—tells us where we and other objects are in space. This spatial information allows us to respond with a wide range of behaviors, from climbing stairs to reading the words on a page. The second path—the ventral path—enables us to identify what objects are.

The ventral and dorsal pathways act independently. However, for us to construct an accurate internal model of the world we live in, the two systems also need to complement each other. When they do, the result is normal behavior. When they don't, people can experience anything from minor learning problems to full-blown breakdowns such as those Ned suffered.

. . . .

In Ned's case, as in Peter's, we were able to address a visual perceptual problem that had led over the years to symptoms severe enough to be labeled as mental illness or emotional instability. We were delighted by the changes we saw in both patients, but saddened to think about the time they had spent suffering unnecessarily. Had they received therapy earlier, they would have been spared years of trauma.

And here is something important to know: it is almost never *too* early to begin addressing a visual perceptual problem. For example, one therapist who once worked for me became anxious when her first child didn't sit up at the typical age. After observing him, I placed a pair of disruptive base-down ambient prisms on him. (I'll talk later about how these prisms affect vision.) The resulting change in his visual perception normalized his vestibulo-ocular reflex, and he immediately sat up—much to everyone's delight.

When we diagnose problems early like this, we put development back on track. As a result, we can prevent learning and emotional problems from occurring, or reverse these problems before they become severe—as my next story shows.

Jane's story

Jane was in first grade when I first saw her. According to the school's paperwork, Jane's visual acuity was less than 20/40 in each eye. But I learned much more about Jane's vision just by watching her in action.

When Jane arrived for her appointment she was anxious, which is exactly what I'd expect from a six-year-old entering a doctor's office. But I also noticed that she couldn't or wouldn't make eye contact and that she kept looking at the floor. When I followed her into the exam room, she walked head-down and tilted to the right, and her gait veered to the left. She also touched the wall as she entered the room.

Immediately, the issue of orientation appeared on my radar. When you can't orient visually to your world, you usually fall back on your sense of touch—just as Jane did when she touched the wall. And when you don't know where you are in relationship to everything around you, you can't stand straight or walk straight.

I tested Jane's ability to read the entire eye chart, and I got the same result as the school—20/40 in each eye. But then I did something they hadn't done: I reduced the chart to a single horizontal line.

When I did that, Jane easily identified letters on the 20/25 line. And when I isolated a single letter at a time, she could identify the letters on the 20/20 line.

That test and others showed me that Jane's problem didn't lie in the hardware (neurological structure) of her eyes. Instead, it lay in the software (perceptual processing) of her brain.

Clearly, Jane had difficulty tracking with her eyes. Her brain had adapted by causing her to focus on a small area at a time—what we call "tunnel vision." As a result, however, she suffered a severe loss of depth perception.

Because of her tunnel vision, Jane had to move her eyes excessively to read or even to move around. She substituted words for the ones she couldn't see. And she often suffered from fatigue and headaches as a result of the stress stemming from her impaired perception.

According to her mom, Jane preferred to stay in her room rather than playing with other kids outside. She showed symptoms of social anxiety as well as "spatial anxiety," a term

I use to describe the stress that people with visual perceptual problems experience when exploring their environment.

As I tested Jane further, I found that she had balance and gait issues stemming from delays in establishing a body schema (something I'll discuss shortly). These delays, and her resulting problems in spatial orientation and organization, also explained why she tended to write lower-case letters backwards.

I put a visual management program in place, and Jane responded beautifully. She's now headache-free, no longer tired, and reading at the top of her class. Her mother reports that while Jane hated to leave the house before, it's now hard to get her to come back inside when she's playing with her friends. She acts and plays just like other children her own age, she's hitting her developmental milestones on target, and she's on course to lead a happy and successful life.

Changing lives by enhancing spatial orientation and organization

As a result of therapy, the three patients I've talked about in this chapter achieved a higher level of functioning in two different areas: spatial *orientation* and spatial *organization*. The level of efficiency each of us achieves in the orientation to and organizing of space dictates our success (or failure) in achieving a normal relationship, both biologically and psychologically, with our world. Here is a look at each crucial skill.

1. SPATIAL ORIENTATION

Are you sitting upright right now, or lying down? Are your shoulders tilted? If so, a little or a lot—and in which direction?

Is your head (or your hand, or your foot) moving? If so, how fast is it moving, and in what direction?

Your mind can answer these questions because you have the ability to orient yourself in space—that is, to constantly monitor your own position and movement. Most people assume that we're born with this ability, but in reality it develops as we interact with our environment.

To orient ourselves in space, we need to develop a *body schema*—a mental model of our body that allows us to organize the information we get from our senses so we can constantly update our position. Observe a young baby, and you'll see her developing her body schema as she discovers herself by moving parts of her body and using her eyes: "Where is my hand?" "What are my fingers doing in space?" "Where does my hand stop and the outside world begin?"

Three systems work together to create our awareness of our position and movement in space: our *visual* system, our *proprioceptive* system (which provides feedback from our muscles, tendons, and skin), and our *vestibular* system (see section entitled "The vestibular system" below). This awareness develops slowly as we age, and it makes a big leap rather suddenly between the ages of seven and eight.

As children refine their body schema, they also master new skills, including rolling over, sitting up, crawling, standing, walking, and running. Most children can achieve these skills fairly easily because *the eyes are leading the mind.* In other words, these children's brains are smoothly and unconsciously processing information from their eyes, allowing them to maintain a correct body schema. At any given moment, they can tell exactly where their arms, legs, and head are located.

Sometimes, however, problems arise in the brain's visual software. When this happens, the mind needs to step in and take control in order to solve the problem—and this, in turn, leads to delays which persist throughout life.

I like to use the analogy of a highway. If the highway is smooth and straight, you can drive down it quickly and easily. But if it's blocked by an accident or a fallen tree, you'll need to slow down to a crawl or maybe even take an indirect route on some side streets. As a result, it's going to be more difficult, and it's going to take you longer to get to where you're going.

Similarly, when the mind needs to lead the eyes, more processing needs to occur before you can take action. As a result, a time lag occurs—and that lag makes it more difficult to correctly orient and stabilize yourself in space. This makes your environment less predictable and more confusing, and it's why people with visual processing impairments find it difficult or even impossible to cope with the demands of their world.

. . . .

The vestibular system: a key player in creating a body schema

It's easy to understand why visual and proprioceptive feedback can help you to know where you are in space. But what does your vestibular system have to do with it?

The vestibular system, which is part of the labyrinth in the inner ear, is responsible for sensing the movements of your head. Signals from the vestibular system drive a reflex called the vestibulo-ocular reflex (VOR). This reflex stabilizes images on the retinas of your eyes when you move your head, by causing your eyes to move in the opposite direction. Disorders of vestibular function result in an abnormal VOR, causing you to get incomplete and sometimes misleading information about where your body is in space.

Vestibular symptoms don't occur in isolation. Patients may complain of everything from dizziness to motion sickness, and an abnormal VOR can express itself in different ways in different patients.

In my opinion, symptoms like this result from a conflict between visual and vestibular perception. This results in an illusion of self-motion, leading to a loss of spatial orientation and postural control.

. . . .

2. SPATIAL ORGANIZATION

While spatial *orientation* refers to our internal development of a body schema, spatial *organization* refers to our ability to organize the objects and events in our world in relationship to each other, ourselves, and other people. For example, good spatial organization allows us to hit a baseball (because we know our location and can swing accurately toward the location of the ball), or to drive safely in traffic (because we know the position of our own car, the cars around us, and the cars parked to the side).

Spatial organization originates with the body schema, which provides a three-dimensional reference point of "self." Once we know where we are in space, we can begin to tell left from right and understand what's above or below us. We can tell which direction a dog or a car is moving in, and how quickly it's moving toward or away from us. And we can learn how to identify alphabet letters and how to read sentences from left to right.

If visual perceptual delays prevent us from developing good spatial organization skills, we can fail to develop a good sense of laterality (left–right) and direction. When this happens, we'll have problems in knowing where objects in our world are located in relation to our bodies. We'll be clumsy, we'll read poorly, and we'll struggle to do even simple activities.

Peter, Ned, and Jane are clear examples of how crucial functional spatial orientation and organization are to our survival. When these skills are intact, we live and learn. When they are not, we must struggle to learn to live. In fact, I can often predict, based on a person's spatial orientation and organization skills, how well that person is doing in life—academically, professionally, socially, and emotionally. The greater the person's deficits, the more he or she will need to fight just to survive.

But the good news, as I will discuss in this book, is that these deficits are subject to reprogramming—not just in childhood, but at any stage of life. In effect, we can rewrite the brain's visual software, and by rewriting that software, we can change a life. In the remainder of this section, I will talk about the techniques and tools I use to accomplish this goal.

2 THE POWER OF A LENS

Vision begins with light stimulating our eyes, which are optical transformers that form images on the retina. These images, in turn, are received by the brain, which interprets (processes) them so we can formulate thoughts and plan actions.

To interact successfully with our world, this system needs to work swiftly and dynamically. This can happen only if our mind creates a stable perception of space even as our eyes, head, and body are moving.

Most of the patients I see have lost their ability to do this. To help them regain this ability, I use ambient yoked prisms. Ambient prism lenses (which alter peripheral vision) are worn in standard eyeglass frames, and they look exactly the same as conventional eyeglasses. However, they incorporate wedge prisms rather than standard refractive prisms. Conventional prisms alter central light rays, while ambient prisms alter peripheral light rays.

Ambient yoked prisms, like all lenses, transform light energy—but these special lenses play a unique role in vision therapy. In this chapter, I explain how I discovered these powerful tools and why they are the cornerstone of the therapy I provide.

My "aha" moment

In 1972, I became aware that the lenses I prescribed for focal vision problems were correcting sight but not fully correcting my patients' visual impairments. Many of my patients at that time were over 40 and had age-related focusing problems (presbyopia). When they began wearing their glasses, they'd tell me that they could see clearly—but they'd also say that they had trouble reading for long periods or keeping their place on the page. In addition, they complained about experiencing fatigue, headaches, or even nausea when they did activities requiring close-up vision. While their glasses made things clear, these patients still couldn't process movement and depth.

Many of these patients were wearing conventional lenses with a single-prism design to correct "sight" (identification) issues such as myopia, hyperopia, astigmatism, or improper ocular alignment—all hardware problems. But I realized that I also needed to address their neural organization.

I was familiar back then with the work of Bruce Wolff, a Cincinnati optometrist who used yoked prisms as a vision training tool. He was using large-magnitude yoked prisms on a temporary basis to disrupt patients' vision, thus forcing them to change the way they processed visual information so they could make better sense of their surroundings (a concept I'll discuss later).

My concept was to use low-magnitude yoked prisms, not to disrupt but to guide the actions of the eyes so they could lead the brain. It was an "aha" moment in my professional life. The results were exciting, and before long my colleagues nicknamed me "the yoked prism man."

Once I discovered the power of prisms in treating vision problems, I was able to develop a clinical approach to help many of my patients. This model, which took many years to create, involves applying yoked prisms of equal magnitude and direction to both eyes. This is a paradigm shift from the conventional use of prism lenses in one eye.

Brain mapping and single prisms versus yoked prisms

There are three steps to visually integrating mind, body, and world. First, we receive visual stimuli via our eyes. Next, our mind organizes this information into "visual maps" so we can make sense of what we're seeing. And finally, our body acts on the information.

For these three steps to occur properly, our eyes must be "yoked." That is, the brain must direct the eyes to move simultaneously in the correct directions (just like a team of yoked oxen). When the eyes become unyoked, the information we receive becomes unstable and our behavior, in turn, becomes disordered.

In my experience, I find that a single prism de-yokes the visual process, and that this de-yoking interferes with normal mapping. This can actually exacerbate the problems of a person with visual dysfunction, worsening symptoms such as abnormal posture, tunnel vision, attention problems, and anxiety. For example, most practitioners I know say that using single prisms to align the eyes as a treatment for a vertical imbalance often increases the deviation rather than lessening it.

Yoked prisms, on the other hand, facilitate the natural biological mapping process by transforming the light entering the eyes and encouraging the eyes to move together in a uniform manner. As a result, these prisms cause a remapping of a person's visual surroundings that improves spatial organization and orientation. In addition, low-magnitude yoked prisms allow patients to achieve perceptual constancy by reducing the number of eye movements, head movements, and body movements they need to make in order to collect information.

Conventional lenses, which address the hardware of the eye, immediately help patients with refractive errors see more clearly. However, these lenses rarely change these patients' actions. In reality, the clarity with which people can identify objects in their world has a limited influence on their behavior.

Yoked prisms, conversely, rarely change clarity. But as the following patient's letter shows, these lenses—which address the software of the brain—can dramatically change behavior.

(Note: as the following letter implies, the change is immediate when patients put on the prisms. When they take off the lenses, their perception will revert. However, with therapy, their perceptions will consolidate and their adaptations will persist.)

Dear Dr. Kaplan,

Tim suggested I wait a few weeks to send you a progress report but the glasses have not yet controlled my impatience and I decided to write you in the first flush of excitement.

You must already know what a relief it was to find a doctor who understood my complaints. Thirty-some years of being told by the "finest" ophthalmologists that I had "20/20" vision while I complained of severe discomfort had not convinced me I was crazy, but I was beginning to believe I was incurable.

I'm afraid my excitement after your initial examination created expectations of a miraculous cure and today, when I first put on my new glasses, I must confess I expected to be instantly able to jump higher, run faster, lose 15 pounds, and win the Miss America competition. Needless to say, I was momentarily disappointed.

As a matter of fact, as I tarried in the Tarrytown shops, putting on and taking off the glasses, and then drove, in blinding sunlight, to Newark, my disappointment was more than momentary. By the time I got to [my husband] Tim's office, I had decided to give myself a chance to get accustomed to the changes and I relaxed a bit.

We left Newark and drove to Philadelphia. A few miles from home I made a startling observation. My eyes had been open for the whole trip without any conscious effort on my part to keep them open. My facial muscles were relaxed for the first time in years, and my eyes didn't hurt! In addition, Tim's driving didn't make me nervous and when I took the wheel to try my night driving, the oncoming lights didn't bother me at all.

Meanwhile, I must express my extreme gratitude to you and to all the people with whom you worked to develop this approach to visual problems. Words cannot adequately convey my delight, amazement, relief, and pleasure in being visually symptom-free for the first time I can remember.

Sincerely,
JB

Initially, JB's husband, Tim, a physician, wasn't as impressed as his wife. In fact, he was highly skeptical. However, after watching her transformation and then receiving prism lenses himself, Tim wrote the following letter to the doctor who'd referred JB to me:

I was, as you know, a doubter, a skeptic of the profession. But I must admit now to being a believer. While the following evidence is mostly anecdotal, I offer my credentials, not only as a long-suffering patient, but as a man trained in science.

Item: JB says—and I am quite aware—my eyes do not dart every second while I am trying to concentrate or talk to someone.

Item: I am able to concentrate in a way I have not done in 10 or 15 years. I can read now, sometimes for two or three hours at a time. Moreover, my attention span, which used to be about 15 microseconds before I darted to something else (this would occur in the course of conversation, reading, working—what have you), has now focused, such that I can actually maintain attention on one item at a time. I was miserable before, my mind was flying all over the place, flitting like some poor bird in winter over the frozen ground, stopping for an instant before flying on. I can actually finish a sentence now, according to JB.

One crucial key in transforming patients' visual processes is to select the correct prism lenses, because different patients require different interventions. Depending on my patients' needs, I may choose base-up, base-down, base-left, or base-right yoked prisms. Here is how these prisms affect vision.

PRISM TYPE	EFFECT ON PERCEPTION AND PERFORMANCE
BASE-UP	Base-up prisms affect rotation about the horizontal axis in space, rotating the visual level of attention to a lower, closer field of view. This leads to a slight downward tunneling or focusing of one's field of vision. There is a corresponding effect on vergence movements (in which the eyes move inward, as in reading), improving spatial organization, sense of timing, and awareness of depth.

BASE-DOWN	Base-down prisms affect rotation about the horizontal axis in space, rotating the visual level of attention higher and further away. This leads to a slight upward expansion of one's field of vision. There is a corresponding effect on vergence movements, improving spatial organization, sense of timing, and awareness of depth.
BASE-LEFT	Base-left prisms rotate the energy input about the vertical axis, moving attention toward the right field of view. This affects orientation, influencing posture, transport (walking), and vergence eye movements.
BASE-RIGHT	Base-right prisms rotate the energy input about the vertical axis, moving attention toward the left field of view. This affects orientation, influencing posture, transport (walking), and vergence eye movements.

Yoked prisms and illusion versus reality

Both low-magnitude yoked prisms and high-magnitude yoked prisms create perceptual illusions. The real world remains the same, but my patients react to the perceptual illusion.

To understand this, picture yourself watching a 3-D movie or looking at a 3-D picture. You'll react to the illusion—for instance, a monster jumping out of the movie screen, or an image rising up from the page—and not to the reality in front of you.

The difference between the two types of prisms I use is that low-magnitude prism illusions are perceived unconsciously (with little or no awareness of the visual displacement), while large-magnitude illusions are perceived consciously (with obvious awareness of the visual displacement). For example, if I sent you to an art museum with very-low-magnitude yoked prisms, they would enhance your ability to stably perceive the paintings you saw—but you would not be consciously aware of this improvement. If I switched you to large-magnitude yoked prisms, you'd become consciously aware of aberrations of form, color, and depth.

In JB's case, low-magnitude prisms helped her perceive her world more clearly, but she didn't consciously recognize the change. Sometimes, however, I need to hit patients with a hammer—a large application of yoked prism—rather than tickling them with a feather. My approach to treating Martha, a 21-year-old nonverbal woman with autism, is a good example.

When Martha came to my office with her mother, she did something very strange: she entered the room with her eyes closed. In fact, she walked everywhere in my office with her eyes tightly shut.

Martha's previous eye specialist hadn't wanted to deal with this behavior. "When she opens her eyes," he said, "bring her back to my office." But I'm always up for a challenge, which is why I frequently am my patients' court of last appeal.

My guess as I watched Martha was that her visual processing was so unstable that it interfered with her ability to obtain information from her other senses. Her solution was to eliminate the confusing visual input by closing her eyes.

Martha had an expressionless face, her posture was like a mannequin's, and she tightly controlled her movements. Although she didn't speak, she could understand what I said and was able to follow my directions.

I discovered that in new situations, Martha would stand and open her eyes. When I asked her to move, she would close her eyes and accurately walk to where she wanted to be. For example, when I asked her to sit in an exam chair, she opened her eyes. Then she closed them, walked directly to the chair, and sat in it. I realized that Martha had a photographic memory when it came to static images of her surroundings.

Interestingly, I'd worked with a patient much like Martha not long before. Lily also had behaved like a mannequin. Not a hair on her head was out of place, her clothes were perfectly neat, and her mother said her room was always spotless. Her eye and body movements were tightly controlled like Martha's, and although she had language, she wouldn't engage in conversation. She was a great help with household chores, and at other times she just blended in with the scenery.

In Lily's case, I'd initially used large-magnitude disruptive yoked prisms. Her reaction was very positive. In fact, three months into therapy, her mother said, "What did you do to me? Her room is a mess, she's out with her friends, her dress is sloppy—she's a typical teen!"

I decided that the approach that worked for Lily might be ideal for Martha. But in Martha's case, I had the added challenge of her closed eyes.

The answer I came up with was to take her by surprise. I had Martha sit three feet in front of me with her eyes closed. I reached for a fully inflated basketball and threw it softly at her body. When the ball hit her, she became startled and opened her eyes. She looked at me and immediately closed her eyes again. After a few repetitions, Martha realized that she had to allow her eyes to guide her hands in order to defend herself, so she kept her eyes open during the activity.

Next, I placed two chairs 12 feet apart and asked Martha to sit in one of the chairs. Then I instructed her to stand and walk to the other chair. She was able to accomplish the task by opening her eyes and then closing them as she walked. But I had a surprise for her. I took a pair of 20-diopter (high-magnitude) base-left yoked prisms and placed them on her face. (These lenses displace all of the objects in a person's field of vision by 20 degrees to the right.) Martha didn't fuss, but she kept her eyes closed. Then I again asked Martha to walk to the other chair and sit down. She was relaxed, because she'd already succeeded at this task. But this time when she opened her eyes, she created a new photographic memory of the perceptual illusion she saw through the prisms. Her response was to the illusion: she walked in a direction to the right of the chair and ran into a wall. She wasn't hurt, but she was quite startled.

This new experience was an awakening for Martha, and she kept her eyes open as I continued to test her. Unlike JB, Martha was consciously aware of the prisms' effect, and this awareness was highly motivating for her. She was even more motivated when she discovered later that she could catch a ball with low-magnitude prisms that transformed her depth perception and reduced her anxiety when she tracked a target.

. . . .

Prisms and visual adaptation

The term *visual adaptation* refers to how the visual system responds to changes in the environment. To make these continual adjustments, the brain needs to process huge amounts of information quickly—just as computers in a satellite need to constantly make adjustments in order to track, process, and make sense of incoming data.

The transformation caused by ambient yoked prisms immediately creates subtle or sometimes dramatic changes in visual adaptation that cause a patient to respond with both conscious and unconscious alterations in performance and perception. I can observe and measure these changes and determine how consistent they are. This allows me to decide when and if ambient yoked prisms need to be prescribed, changed, maintained, or removed.

. . . .

Progressing from illusion to real-life motivation

The rapid positive changes that ambient prism lenses cause are hugely motivating for my patients, and they often move quickly from skepticism to delight. Sean, a ten-year-old with academic issues and behavioral problems, is a good example.

Sean's mom had taken him from doctor to doctor with little luck. When she told him that she was taking him to see me, Sean said that under no condition would he wear glasses. His mom told him, "This doctor is different. He may be able to suggest a solution to help you read more easily—and maybe he can make you an even better ball player."

When I examined Sean, I found that his eye movements prevented him from capturing a stable image on his retinas. In addition, he had problems with depth perception.

I said to Sean, "Mom tells me that you're a pretty good ball player." He answered, "I'm able to keep up."

I asked if we could play catch. Sean smiled and answered, "Why not?"

When I threw the ball to Sean, he jumped to the side and reached out his hand to the left and caught the ball. Each time I tossed the ball, the same thing happened. I said, "Your form is different from most kids'. Do you know why you developed that method of catching?"

Sean said, "My brother is older, and he's a good player. I wanted to keep up."

I said, "Let's try something different." I placed low-magnitude two-diopter yoked prisms on him, and his shoulders immediately dropped and appeared to relax. Then I said, "Try it again." Sean stood his ground, reached out, and caught the ball. Now it was his turn to say, "Let's try that again." And again, he caught the ball easily in a normal way.

Sean asked me, "If I get these lenses, how long will I need them?" I said that, in my experience, it would take 10 to 12 months.

Without hesitation, he replied, "Let's try them out."

Moving from neural changes to permanent behavioral changes

Patients often show immediate changes when I place yoked prism lenses on them. (I think of this as "instant gratification.") However, these lenses aren't meant to be worn permanently, like glasses for near-sightedness or other focal problems. Instead, they're generally a temporary tool to "capture" an improvement in behavior that we can consolidate with therapy.

In fact, one of the major differences between conventional lenses and yoked prisms is that conventional lenses, which alter *what we see*, are corrective in nature. In other words, they are designed to correct a permanent hardware problem. Ambient yoked prisms, which control *where we look*, are adaptive in nature. Think of them as training wheels for the brain.

How do I determine when it's time to take these training wheels off? I look for changes in patients' behavior, performance, and visual adaptation—and I also listen to what patients tell me. And sometimes, my patients surprise me.

Stan, a 45-year-old dentist, was one of these patients. At his first appointment, Stan explained to me that his specialty was dental reconstruction. He spent one or two hours each session working in a patient's mouth, an extremely close-up task. Although he wore lenses for presbyopia (blurred near vision), he still found that he developed visual fatigue earlier and earlier in sessions, and this affected his sight. At the start of a session, he told me, the patient's mouth would be clear. After twenty minutes, it would start to blur, and finally he would reach a point where he couldn't see well enough to do his work.

My examination showed that Stan had tunnel vision, his depth perception was questionable, and his gaze stability deteriorated over time, requiring excessive eye movements. I asked him, "When you work inside a patient's mouth, how much of the patient's face do you see?" He told me, "At the start I can see out to their ears. I end up seeing only the upper or lower part of the patient's mouth."

A program including ambient yoked prism lenses and movement awareness worked well for Stan. Six months into the program, his visual perceptual profile had improved so much that I felt the prism lenses might push him in the wrong direction. I discussed my findings with him and he said, "My energy when I'm working is at a level where I'm totally comfortable."

I prescribed a new pair of glasses for Stan, without the prisms. Two days later, I got a call from Stan: "Put the prisms back." The numbers were there, but Stan still needed time to adjust to the changes in his vision. It took him another few months to be ready to let go of the prism lenses.

So there's no exact moment when I know the lenses have done their job. It takes as long as it takes—but eventually the training wheels come off. And when they do, my patients are ready to see their world in a new and better way.

. . . .

Vision therapy: the age myth

One fact that surprises many of my fellow professionals is that yoked prisms work for adults like Martha and Stan as well as for children like Sean. There's a misconception that visual processes aren't sufficiently plastic for treatment to be effective for older children or adults. But I have successfully used yoked prisms to treat everyone from infants to senior citizens. My experience is consistent with scientific research showing that the brain's sensory maps are generally established early in normal development but remain somewhat plastic throughout life.

. . . .

What I've learned from my patients

It took a long time for me to understand what my patients who were wearing yoked prism lenses were telling me about the changes they experienced in both performance and perception. Over time, I began to grasp what was happening as I witnessed similar responses over and over again. Here are some examples:

- One woman told me that the room immediately seemed larger and brighter.

- A teenager said he could read faster and with greater comprehension.

- A 65-year-old Ph.D. at Columbia University remarked when I threw a ball for him to catch, "Oh my God, it's the first time in 25 years that I don't feel the tightness in my chest."

- When I placed high-magnitude prisms on a six-year-old, mostly nonverbal child during a workup, she stood up and started to dance and every expletive I'd ever heard came out of her mouth. When I tried to remove the prisms, she grabbed onto them and started to scream, "My eyes, my eyes!"

Eventually, I came to realize that conventional lenses correct problems that involve viewing the world in 2-D (for instance, identifying a letter on a page), while yoked prisms address problems that involve viewing the world in 3-D (for instance, understanding where a moving object is in space). Prisms affected my patients immediately and dramatically because for the first time in years—or in some cases, the first time in their lives—these patients were able to see the world in three dimensions.

Before discovering the power of prisms, I had focused solely on skills training, which led to better performance but didn't change perception. Successful adaptation, I learned, requires *both* the application of yoked prisms to change patients' perception *and* new experiences to change their performance.

Combining these two approaches—prisms and training— empowers my patients to see their world accurately in 3-D. As a result, they can process more information in less time. Mind, body, and world come into balance, increasing knowledge and decreasing stress. I call this the *perceptual* model, and it can be summed up in this simple formula:

space × *time* = *knowledge*

In this model, *space* relates to the external world and *time* involves the internal processing we need to perform in order to gain information from this world and process it in our mind. The more quickly my patients can do this, the more knowledge they can acquire. And the more knowledge they can acquire, the more successfully they can navigate their world.

The path to this improved performance begins with selecting the correct prism lenses for each patient. And making the right choice requires an ability to "read" each patient—something I discuss in the next chapter.

3

THE IMPORTANCE OF
READING PEOPLE

Tests and diagnostic equipment can give vision professionals a vast amount of data about their patients' visual problems. But in my experience, equally important clues come from watching patients move around my office.

This is why I add another dimension to my evaluations, going beyond standard tests and adding pre- and post-tasks to identify patients' symptoms and analyze how they respond to ambient yoked prisms. For example, if a patient's head posture tilts left, I will use base-left ambient yoked prisms to see if the person's posture becomes erect while standing or walking.

There are many benefits to "reading" a patient as the person performs tasks without and then with prisms. First, both the patient and I get instant feedback about what the person's issues truly are. Second, I can confirm which type and direction of prism I need to use. And third, patients become highly motivated to proceed with therapy when they see how dramatically their performance changes with the application of prisms.

Here's a quick illustration. A 62-year-old woman, watching her husband's evaluation, asked, "Can you help me?" She told me she was born with her right leg one inch shorter than her left leg, which led to pain in her groin area every time she walked.

I asked her to walk to the mirror on the opposite side of the room. I noticed that as she walked, her right leg appeared to drag while her left leg rose. I placed two-diopter base-right prisms on her, knowing that this would cause her to shift her weight slightly to her left side. Then I asked her to walk to the mirror again. When she reached the mirror, she turned and said, "This is the first time I have walked free of pain in my groin." The transformation she underwent as a result of the prisms was preconscious, but she could consciously recognize the results when she looked in the mirror and when she realized that her pain was gone. As a result, she was highly motivated to begin therapy herself.

To me, results like this demonstrate why it is crucial not to view symptoms as a *problem*, as most vision specialists do. Instead, we need to view symptoms as a clue to the *solution*.

As I see it, patients' actions—no matter how odd those actions may seem—are their attempts to solve problems, either inherited or acquired. In other words, a symptom is an external solution to an internal disorganization of the brain.

Unlike other vision specialists, I don't examine the visual system in isolation but instead view the individual as a whole. The "software" issues that cause visual processing deficits will reveal themselves as disorders of body movements, eye movements, and depth perception. Also, I don't view a patient's responses as "right" or "wrong," but rather as clues to the person's mental information processing. Finally, I look at those responses as the interaction of mind, body, and task.

Typically, optometrists or ophthalmologists take a history first, and then complete a comprehensive examination and come up with a diagnosis. But that's not what I do. Instead, I "read" each patient's posture and movement and profile the person's behavior. Then I say, "Here's how I see this behavior and how it impacts learning, social interaction, and posture." Finally, I follow up with formal testing to measure the patient's performance. In this process, I focus not only on hardware problems such as far-sightedness, but also—and even more importantly—on software issues. Here are some real-life examples of the issues my exams can reveal.

Dwight: the class clown

Dwight, a 15-year-old high school sophomore, constantly disrupted his class by clowning around. When his teacher reprimanded him for his behavior, he'd look anywhere but at her as she was speaking.

One day, out of frustration, she raised her voice and said, "Look at me when I talk to you." His response was, "If I look at you, I can't hear you." Throwing up her hands in despair, she sent him to the principal's office.

Soon after that, Dwight's mother brought him to see me. The question for me when he entered my office was: Is Dwight really just a disobedient kid, or does he have an underlying delay in development?

To answer this question, I performed my standard three-part evaluation. Here are the steps in this lengthy evaluation:

- *Visual Behavior Profiling:* The tests I have patients perform at this stage allow me to evaluate the degree of freedom they experience in mind and body as they respond to the demands of the world. Over time, I've learned that patients exhibit recognizable patterns on the Visual Skills Test (a modification of the Gesell Keystone Battery) and Kaplan Star Test (see Appendix I). These patterns allow me to profile people's information-processing ability and their visual organization and orientation skills. In short, these tests differentiate between "normal" (ordered) and "abnormal" (disordered) responses.

- *Qualitative Behavior Analysis:* This part of the exam involves a group of activities such as ball play and figure/ground activities without and with yoked prisms. This analysis answers two questions for me. The first is, "Can we change performance?" The second is, "Can we change perception?" In addition, my analysis informs me about the magnitude and direction of prism needed for guiding changes.

- *Quantitative Visual Analysis:* In this exam, I measure visual acuity, refractive error, and ocular alignment, as well as screening for eye disease. This is similar to the exam that most vision specialists do.

Dwight's exam revealed a profile of symptoms indicating that he had poor control of his eye movements. This impacted his depth perception and interfered with his ability to maintain eye contact.

Dwight wasn't the type to force himself to pay attention. He was a *flighter* rather than a *fighter*. In other words, it was much easier for him to escape or avoid a problem than to meet it head-on. Therefore, I knew he would find reading stressful, have trouble keeping his place, and need to re-read.

As I continued to test Dwight, I made several additional observations about his behavior:

- He avoided eye contact, a further clue to his depth perception issues. When we stood and faced each other, his head kept turning and his gaze constantly shifted to avoid my eyes. In development, a child first learns to attend to vertical space cues, then to horizontal space cues, and finally to depth cues. Because of Dwight's delays, his attention to sagittal (depth) space failed to develop, making eye contact difficult for him. (By the way, 25 to 30 percent of the population have difficulty attending to sagittal space. Research shows that watching 3-D movies causes people with this problem to become dizzy and have headaches and in some cases stomachaches.)

- While standing, Dwight often rocked from side to side. This told me that he had orientation issues. People who skip steps in learning to orient themselves to their world will often rock side-to-side in order to determine where their body is.

At this point, I needed to confirm my predictions, make Dwight consciously aware of his visual issues, and present a solution to motivate him.

To do this, I used a simple task. First, I placed three letters of equal size (one-inch high) an equal distance apart at Dwight's eye level. The T and P were the same color, while the O was a different color.

T O P

I asked Dwight to look at the O. "Without moving your eyes off the O," I said, "tell me—are all three letters equally clear? His response was, "No." I asked which letter was the clearest. He replied, "The T is the clearest, and the O is blurry."

Dwight's profile called for yoked base-up prisms. Placing a pair of glasses with only two diopters of prism base-up in each eye, I repeated the question. This time he smiled and said, "They're all clear."

The following drawing illustrates the perceptual change Dwight underwent with the help of the glasses. At first, his eye movements would jump from the left visual field to the right visual field. The ambient prism lenses transformed his perception, so he was able to see a uniform binocular field as shown below.

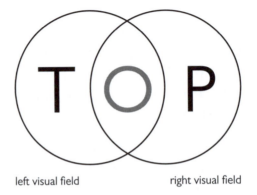

left visual field · · · · · · · · · · · · · · right visual field

Dwight was excited by the effects of the prism lenses, and he was highly motivated to continue. But I said, "Let's do one more thing." This time, I asked him to read without and with the prisms. He found that the prisms made him feel stronger and less tense. His reading was smooth, and his comprehension improved.

Immediately, he turned to me and said, "Okay, you got me. Where do we go from here?"

· ·

Clinical pearl: spotting poor depth perception

Our brains use a variety of clues, gained from both binocular vision and monocular vision, to create our three-dimensional world. When this process fails, patients exhibit a variety of symptoms:

- When they read, they may re-read sentences, lose their place and start over again, or voice the words under their breath. They may also develop headaches or eye strain.

- When they play sports, they may pull their head back and catch the ball close to their body because their timing is off.

- If they try their hand at art, their works may look "flat."

- Socially and emotionally, they will feel constrained and stressed because they need to focus much of their attention on sorting out a confusing world.

Abraham: The case of the disappearing myopia

Dwight was a *flighter* who ran away from his vision problems rather than confronting them. But Abraham, a 16-year-old high school student, was a *fighter*. He compressed his field of view into tunnel vision, using excessive eye movements to maintain single vision so he could obtain information about depth and movement in his environment. While this allowed him to compensate for his visual deficits, it led to a new set of problems.

Abraham entered my office wearing glasses prescribed for him four months earlier because he couldn't see the blackboard at school. His doctor had determined that Abraham had myopia (near-sightedness), a visual defect in which objects at a distance appear blurry because their images focus in front of the retina rather than on it. The new lenses gave Abraham clarity and a visual acuity of 20/20 in each eye.

That was Abraham's first eye examination and his first pair of glasses. The reason his parents asked for a second opinion from me was that Abraham still had problems. In fact, he now felt more stress when reading than he had before he wore the glasses.

This immediately raised a key question: Was Abraham's myopia structural or functional? The difference is crucial, because the two types of myopia require two different treatments.

Structural myopia is inherited, just as genes dictate height. This type of myopia can worsen as a child grows and the length of the eye increases (usually until 14 to 15 years of age), thus increasing the refractive error. Structural myopia is usually of high magnitude, and the treatment is to simply increase the magnitude of the lens.

Functional myopia, on the other hand, is acquired as a person interacts with the world. It's usually associated with near-point stress—for instance, heavy reading. Functional myopia is usually of low magnitude.

· ·

Functional myopia: what the research shows

Two studies reveal the impact of everyday life on myopia. In the first study, researchers found that Eskimo children rarely exhibited myopia. When they started attending school, however, more than half developed myopia. A second study of Harvard students found that 20 percent were myopic in their freshman year, while a full 80 percent were myopic by their senior year.

· ·

In Abraham's case, he was able to attain 20/30 visual acuity without any glasses. This strengthened my suspicion that his myopia was acquired and was a product of near-point stress.

When I asked Abraham to track a moving target from left to right while sitting, he performed normally. (This form of eye tracking, in which both eyes move in the same direction, is called *version* movement.) However, when I asked him to follow the target as it moved toward him—an action called *vergence* movement, in which the eyes both turn inward—he became stressed and his right eye turned in further than his left eye. Testing at near point showed that Abraham had tunnel vision, and other tests revealed depth perception issues that affected his focusing and led to ocular spasm. The result was myopia and visually-induced stress.

It was easy for me to demonstrate Abraham's problems to him. I asked him if he was a ball player, and he said no. I said, "Let me show you why not."

I had him stand about four feet from me. Then I took a ball and tossed it at him. He responded by blinking his eyes—a sign of fear—and his body moved backward.

Then I asked him to sit in a chair. Again, I threw a ball at him. This time his hands went out to meet the ball and he held his head steady, although I could still see that he felt stressed.

I explained to Abraham that his greater impairment when he tried to catch the ball while standing indicated delays in spatial orientation. Then I placed ambient yoked prisms on him and threw the ball at him again. Both when sitting and when standing, his performance appeared perfectly normal.

This demonstration made Abraham conscious of his issues with orientation and depth perception. I told him that what he'd just witnessed wasn't magic but rather his mind's ability to reprogram. I also explained that to make this change permanent, he'd need a visual management program.

Abraham was highly motivated, especially when I told him how visual management could improve both his reading and his ability to play sports. "A bonus," I said, "is that it's possible that the clarity of your sight may return and you won't need glasses."

My examination had revealed that Abraham's myopia wasn't structural but rather was a behavioral response to his primary problem: poor gaze stability. He wasn't able to tell where things were in space, resulting in stress, particularly during near-point activities like reading.

The chief goal of Abraham's treatment was for him to achieve relaxed attention, allowing him to process more information in less time. One key component of my treatment plan was a procedure I call "defocusing." In this approach, I intentionally reduced Abraham's ability to focus his eyes by applying +5.00 lenses. To understand the effect of this approach, think about your early childhood when you had perfect vision and occasionally tried on older people's high-prescription glasses, causing everything to become blurry.

Defocusing reduced Abraham's ability to identify objects in space, initiating a "letting go" of the controls his mind put in place. This in turn increased his dependence on his spatial world—that is, his ambient visual pathways—giving him more information about *where* things were.

During therapy, Abraham's mind had to learn to control his motor system in its search for information. This is important because the mind is capable of "motor equivalence," which means that it can choose many paths of action as it searches for and processes information. Before therapy, Abraham's mind had chosen a less efficient path. Therapy became his GPS, giving him better directions to the highway so he could speed up his trip.

As a result, his prescription went from two diopters of myopia at baseline to one diopter at the start of therapy and zero at the end of the program. His enhanced visual skills also allowed him to perform at the top of his class and to enjoy sports.

Patrick: the high-IQ kid who couldn't read

Patrick's mother brought him to my office when he was seven years old. He had an IQ of 140, yet he found reading excruciatingly difficult. Patrick's performance showed that he was able to localize (fixate his eyes on a target). He also was able to fuse the images from both eyes.

My first clue about Patrick's visual processing disorder came during a 2-D test in which each eye sees a different picture and the brain has to unify these into a single picture. One eye sees an arrow pointing up, while the other eye sees a single row of numbers.

My assistant asked Patrick, "Is the arrow steady or moving?" His reply was, "Moving." The assistant then asked, "To what number is it moving?" At the near point, the correct answer is from 7 to 9. Patrick started at 2 and moved to 7.

This clearly showed me that Patrick was in trouble. It meant that although he aimed his eyes correctly, he couldn't sustain his gaze, so the two images did not converge into one image. Instead, he'd alternated his eye movements from one picture to the other.

Patrick's alternating eye movements prevented him from capturing a stable picture on his retina. As a result, eye movement was stressful for him, which is why he avoided reading. In addition, his inability to perceive depth caused him to experience dizziness, headaches, and stomachaches.

The Kaplan Star Test (see Appendix I), which examines the function of the ambient visual pathways, offered more clues. When Patrick did the test at near point, the results revealed a pattern of disorganization, tunnel vision, and orientation difficulties.

I reviewed the findings and escorted Patrick into the examination room. As he entered, I studied his posture, gait, and facial expression. He was looking down, his shoulders were up, and his eyes were squinting. To a professional who can read people, this posture says that a patient's field of view is a static 2-D field rather than a dynamic 3-D.

Overall, Patrick had trouble organizing and orienting to his space world. As a result, he saw a tunnel of the world as he moved from far to near. Under visual stress, such as when reading, he had double vision. And his recovery (his return to single vision after experiencing double vision) also took too long.

To adapt, Patrick created habits that masked the stress he experienced. Because of this, he could appear normal. But the amount of energy he had to expend left him breathless and anxious.

Patrick had 20/20 acuity and his ocular health was good. To a doctor who merely looked at test results, he would look visually "normal." But his delays in orientation and organization when he interacted with his surroundings left him struggling. He had a poor body schema, balance issues, and little ability to select effective motor responses to what he saw.

Patrick's vision therapy program involved disruption and reintegration. As he underwent therapy, his posture normalized, and he became able to pay attention in a relaxed way. At one point, he remarked, "Why can't I just wear these lenses forever? They make me feel so good."

Jim: the teacher with headaches

Jim was a 40-year-old teacher who had trouble reading. Looking at books or his students' papers gave him a headache, and he had trouble understanding what he read. He assumed that his problems were age-related, since he'd previously loved reading and had found it easy.

A trip to the eye doctor resulted in a reading prescription and a pair of glasses. However, Jim's symptoms persisted. Then a colleague mentioned that he'd had similar issues and had become symptom-free after getting yoked prisms for reading.

A visit to my office confirmed that Jim needed plus (magnifying) lenses. These made things clearer for him, but he still had poor gaze stability. Observing his eye movements when he read, I could see that his pursuit movements (the eye movements he used to follow the text) were adequate. However, reading also requires a *vergence* movement—turning the eyes in for near-point vision—and Jim had difficulty with this.

Rather than telling Jim how yoked prism lenses would impact his reading, I chose another approach. I stood in front of him and asked him to make eye contact. When he did, I observed that he alternated his glance as he looked at my eyes: first left, then right. This told me that Jim used excessive eye movements to find the print when reading. This led to fatigue, headaches, and other symptoms.

As I'd done with Dwight, I placed three equal-sized letters at eye level on a board in front of Jim—T, O, and P—spacing them equal distances apart. First, I told Jim to look at the O without moving his eye. I asked him, "Are the letters equally clear?" His response was that the T and P were clearer than the O. I placed base-up yoked prisms on him and repeated the task. This time, he said the letters were all equally clear.

Jim's issue wasn't visual clarity. Instead, it was timing. It took him too long to redirect his visual field so he could perceive the words on the page. He also had trouble with figure–ground organization, attending to ground (the background, such as the full page of a book) at the expense of figure (the individual words).

Although Jim's problems related to his near vision, I knew he'd also have issues when he drove a car. I asked him if he had trouble driving at night, and he answered that he was getting a bit anxious. Night driving requires gaze stability, because you need to know where you are and where objects are in relation to you. Jim's system had tunneled in, and he compensated by attending to focal tasks—telling him *what* he saw, but not *where* it was.

I said, "You're probably a fast driver, and I'm guessing you drive in the left lane with your eyes watching the white line." He asked, "How did you know that?" I said that my findings told me that he would experience anxiety and feel a need to get to his destination quickly.

I explained that my examination showed that Jim had an ambient perceptual style, meaning that he preferred ground over figure. However, he had gaze control issues that kept him from forming a stable retinal picture. His mind's solution was to tunnel and perform focally.

Focal viewers prefer linear space, and that is what the white line on the road offers them. However, this comes at the price of filtering out the depth clues. And this, in turn, triggers unconscious anxiety and a need to rush to a destination to stop the anxiety.

Then I asked him another question: "Were you ever a ball player?" Jim said, "I played shortstop for my high school team."

I said, "I'm guessing you were always cuffed when fielding a ground ball." (This means that he wouldn't reach for the ball with his glove but instead responded late and scooped it into his body.) "That's right," he said.

When I talked with Jim about his behavior, it was obvious that he was unaware of the mechanisms controlling his actions. Yet I could see these mechanisms clearly, simply by watching him.

The art and science of reading patients

People typically view other individuals' actions from "inside out"—a psychological interpretation. As a person who treats people from a neurobiological perspective, I view their actions from "outside in"—a physiological perspective.

For example, consider individuals who fail to make eye contact. From a psychological point of view, this may be interpreted as a sign of lying, distraction, submissiveness, or disrespect. But I see this behavior as a means of making sense of information coming from the *outside* in the form of visual stimuli.

As I view it, my patients' initial behaviors are physiological responses to their needs. Later, these patients exhibit psychological responses—for instance, calmness and confidence—as a result of therapy.

My ability to read people fascinates my patients and mystifies my colleagues. However, if professionals stop to think about the process of reading behavior, they'll find that it's not very difficult. They just have to look beyond the standard tests and see the underlying reasons for their patients' behaviors.

This is a skill any professional can master. For instance, I once offered this challenge to a colleague at a conference:

> Imagine that Germaine, an 11-year-old, comes to your office. His mother asks you to evaluate him for behavior and reading problems. You see that Germaine's eye movements are very jumpy when he's tracking a target, his eyes turn too far inward, and he has unstable gaze control. You also see that he has balance issues and drifts when he's walking. From these limited symptoms, can you profile his ability to read?

The doctor thought for a minute, and said that Germaine would have difficulty keeping his place when he read, would re-read words or use his finger to follow the words, and would have comprehension issues. I asked, "Do you think he'd be active in sports?" His answer was, "Probably not."

As we talked, the doctor realized that reading a patient isn't magic. It's simply common sense. The key, as Sherlock Holmes might say, is not just to see—but also to observe.

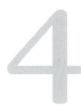

VISUAL MANAGEMENT

From Transforming the Stimulus to Transforming the Behavior

Some people think that transforming the brain's visual software using yoked prism lenses is simply a matter of doing "eye exercises." However, to change a person's visual perception, we need to go beyond simply guiding the person's eye movements.

My model of visual management therapy (VMT) starts with transforming the visual stimulus using prisms and then consolidates the resulting visual perceptual changes by training eye movements. This results in permanent changes in perception, leading to overall improvements in the relationship of mind, body, and world.

Here's an interesting illustration of the power of including prisms in VMT, involving my early experiences in working with patients with schizophrenia. Researchers have known for more than a century that saccades (high-velocity scanning eye movements) are impaired in schizophrenia. In 1990, psychiatrist Frederic Flach invited me to New York University (NYU) to observe researchers who had organized a study to track these abnormal saccades to see if they could be used as a marker for schizophrenia.

In short, the researchers were looking at how *schizophrenia caused abnormal eye movements*. But I knew that *abnormal eye movements could cause many symptoms attributed to schizophrenia*—and that both the abnormal eye movements and the resulting symptoms could be reduced by prism lenses along with a program of visual management.

When the researcher I was observing was finished evaluating his subject, I asked him, "If you were to stop the saccadic eye movement, would that make the subject not schizophrenic?" He looked at me with a startled expression and said, "Why did you ask that?" I replied, "Because stopping abnormal saccadic (jumpy) eye movements is what I do for a living."

As the researcher and I talked, I noticed that his eyes presented a right exotropia (in which the left eye fixates while the right eye turns out). I told him it would be easier to show him what I was trying to explain than to tell him, and I invited him to visit me at my office.

At the office, I asked if he was ever a ball player. He replied that he'd been fearful from an early age when he played ball. I expected him to say this, because his exotropia would prevent accurate depth perception.

I said, "If you can bear with me and subject yourself to catching a wiffle ball, I think I can make myself clear." (A wiffle ball is a light-weight hollow plastic ball.)

I had him sit in a chair with the ball on a string at his chest level, and I tossed it to him. He turned his head and body and was unable to grasp the ball. Then I placed five-diopter base-up ambient yoked prisms on him. I repeated the task, but this time his head and body stayed still, and he reached out and caught the ball. He asked, "What happened?" I responded, "I stopped your saccadic eye movements."

I suggested that we might be able to use ambient yoked prisms to predict his patients' eye movements and resulting behavior. I made up four pairs of five-diopter prism lenses: one base-up, one base-down, one base-right, and one base-left. In addition, I made one plano pair (containing clear, no-prism lenses). I color-coded all of the frames so no one except me could tell which was which.

Three weeks later, Dr. Flach and I returned to the researcher's lab at NYU. I used Dr. Flach as the first patient, asking him to start with the brown glasses. I knew Fred's perceptual style, and I knew that these glasses would disrupt his perception. Fred's eye movement recordings were severely abnormal. Next, I said, "Use the gray pair." This was the plano pair. Fred's second recording was less saccadic. After that, he tried the black pair; I knew it would enhance his performance, and it did. He said this was impressive, but it was probably a "learned response" since it was his third time. So I asked him to repeat the process once more using the brown frame again. This time, his eye movements were quite saccadic.

Unfortunately, the researchers didn't follow up on my demonstration. However, it's one I've repeated many times in my office with patients who have schizophrenia or other mental illnesses. Almost invariably, the correct prisms will cause a dramatic decrease in abnormal saccades and a resulting improvement in behavior and performance.

However, changing eye movements with prisms doesn't mean the battle is won. Once patients can see the world as it really is, they need to unlearn the behaviors they developed to compensate for their visual problems—for instance, over-reliance on other sensory systems such as hearing and touch. In addition, they need to master developmental steps they have skipped.

Overall, a program of VMT must satisfy three goals:

- making patients aware that their performance can change

- moving patients in the direction of relaxed attention

- creating measurable, observable changes.

Accomplishing these goals often requires me to develop novel activities. Here are some examples.

Dylan: balls, balloons, and a rolling pin

At eight years of age, Dylan had issues involving learning, social interaction, and, in particular, sports. His evaluation indicated his issues involved depth perception and spatial orientation. To change his perception, I created a simple and highly motivating program involving balloons and balls.

Three months into Dylan's visual management program, his mother wrote:

> I was particularly impressed with the way Dyl responded to the vision therapy these last two weeks—it was balloon bunting and ball bunting. Dylan has progressed enough that he now has control and breathes in on one hit, out on the other, and he just nails the balloon and ball each time. He's learned how to breathe and move at the same time in the past two weeks and that frees up the neural stream to focus on tracking the ball and tackling it.
>
> Neil took Dylan out and showed him what part of his foot should whack the ball in soccer. He also showed him how to tackle the oncoming opposing soccer player who has the ball: choose left or right; snag it to one side or the other and don't think about advancing until you've got it away from your opponent. He said Dyl was so accurate after that, that he wondered whether he would end up being better than Herschel! (Herschel is the star of all stars in our town, best under-eight player in our league.)
>
> Dyl that good? It's amazing to think how fast he's changing. I lay it all at the feet of VMT. He's a totally

different player than he was this summer. Before, he wasn't able to run. He spent so much energy bouncing up and down that he didn't make much forward progress in his stride. He had so much caution from not knowing where he was in space that he dared not move faster than he could process the new data. Now he's really started to be able to run. Neil said as of yesterday that Dyl's starting to take stutter steps as the ball approached, which he never used to do. His feet used to be planted like tree trunks. It's all coming online, cascading; one thing begetting the next. So fabulous! Neil said he can't wait for Michael (Neil's friend and the boys' soccer coach) to see this change. Dylan loved the VMT exercises so much the last two weeks that he always put more time into them and said to me on the way to VMT yesterday that he doesn't want to ever stop doing the balloon and ball bunting exercises.

The procedure that motivated Dylan so much originated during my examination. At that time, I asked him to catch a ball while standing. When he tried this task, he displayed fear and anxiety as well as impaired performance. I had him sit and lowered the ball so it would again be chest-high, and he showed less fear but still had performance issues.

The next step was to repeat the activity with Dylan seated and wearing two-diopter base-up ambient yoked prisms. This time, he reached out and caught the ball without fear and with good performance and a smile. I asked him to do the same task standing, again with the lenses, and he did it attentively and easily, with no stress.

I knew then that we would introduce balloon and ball bunting early in his therapy to consolidate the performance that the lenses had caused.

First, he started seated, bunting a balloon with a rolling pin while wearing his prism lenses. Then he repeated this task with a baseball-sized wiffle ball, which is faster and smaller. Third, he did the activity sitting and standing with red/green anaglyphs (a red lens in front of his right eye and a green lens in front of his left eye).

In Dylan's case, as his mother's note shows, it took only two weeks for therapy to show astonishing results. And as an added bonus, he enjoyed every minute of it.

Alice: a chopstick task

Alice had issues in visual processing as well as a history of emotional problems, anxiety, and panic attacks. Patients in this situation have two choices when it comes to maintaining a sense of homeostasis with their world: they can either compress their world or alternately view their world via the right and left visual field. In either situation, they reduce the amount of information they need to process, which, in turn, reduces their stress.

Alice preconsciously compressed her visual field, which meant that she needed too much time to interact with the demands of work, running a home, and dealing with family issues. As a result, she was always extremely stressed and anxious. This led to breathing issues, which Alice described as being "thirsty for oxygen."

In Alice's case, I needed to make her unconscious processes conscious. In my experience, the fastest way to do this is to use high-powered prisms (in this case, 20-diopter base-in prisms, another disruptive approach I occasionally use).

Once I determined the appropriate prisms to use, here's the procedure I followed with Alice.

First, I gave Alice red/green lenses to wear under the prisms. Then I asked her to hold chopsticks in each hand and to point them at a nine-inch white balloon ten feet in front of her. She said, "I see two balloons, one red and the other one green." I told her to hold her hands out in front of her and point the sticks at the two balloons she saw, while walking toward them.

As she started to get close, the balloons fused to one white balloon and her chopsticks converged inward. As she moved, I could see her face and body relax. After three or four repetitions of this activity, I gave her a break.

The second part of the procedure repeated the first, using a three-inch white wiffle ball this time. The prism lenses caused increased retinal stimulation, and the red/green lenses gave her additional cues—first revealing her double vision and then her successful fusion (the merging into a single image) and stereopsis (depth perception).

Alice's breathing problems were another interesting aspect of her case. To understand her need for oxygen, it's important to realize that as an infant develops in the womb, there is competition between moving and breathing. If the fetus has trouble organizing the interaction of both moving and breathing, it learns to suppress one at a time. After birth, when competition occurs during development, the mind again chooses. As Alice's visual processing issues resolved, she was able to move more efficiently in space. This freed up more energy and allowed her to breathe more naturally.

Terry: a "pendulum" procedure

Terry was a 27-year-old diagnosed by her therapist as bipolar. She had motion sickness, migraines, and social anxiety, and she told me that there were times she couldn't feel her body.

When I evaluated Terry, I found that she quickly alternated her gaze because she couldn't use both eyes simultaneously in order to process information. I chose to disrupt her behavioral "solutions" by using 20-diopter ambient prism lenses, with one lens set at base-up and the other at base-down. This created double vision.

Initially, I seated Terry with a wiffle ball in front of her on a string at her chest level. I moved the ball like a pendulum across her body and asked her to track the ball. As she followed the ball, I asked her, "How does your jaw feel?" She said, "Tight." Then I asked her, "How does the back of your neck feel?" Again, she said, "Tight."

Next, I placed red/green lenses on her along with the ambient yoked prisms. I adjusted the prisms into the base-up and base-down positions, so that the thick part of the right lens was on the top of the frame and the thick part of the left lens was on the bottom of the frame. (See the description of the intervention at the end of this chapter.) I told her to look at the ball and then asked her, "What do you see?" She answered, "Two balls, one red, one green." I continued to probe with questions about the two balls in order to keep her attention as I observed her body relaxing and her eye tracking becoming smooth.

I also asked her, "How does your jaw feel?" She responded, "Relaxed." I asked about the back of her neck, and she said it was relaxed as well.

Then she volunteered, "This makes me feel better than any of the medications I have been taking."

As a result of this procedure, Terry was able to develop an awareness of where her body was in space. She was so thrilled about the effect of the lenses that she couldn't wait to start her VMT program at home.

The level of performance that my patients reach depends on their mind's ability to "let go" of their established patterns of adaptation and their habitual behavioral solutions as they move from awareness to attention and finally automaticity. Some individuals can permanently accomplish this goal— and when they do, their therapy is done. Others find themselves occasionally reverting to their old patterns, and need an occasional booster. But all of them leave VMT happier, calmer, more confident, and better equipped to take on their world.

Below is a basic intervention we use to help patients achieve a higher level of visual performance. The appropriate response in this exercise is for a patient to see one red and one green ball. If the answer is one ball, the patient is suppressing. When the patient can identify color, placement, and depth, it shows an ability to process more information in less time.

. . . .

Pursuits seated with ball, red/green lenses, and disruption 20 up/20 down and object on head

MATERIALS

I chair

I pair of adjustable prisms (base 20)

I suspended ball

I pair of red and green lenses

I chopstick or pointer, 12 inches long (optional)

I bean bag toy or hat.

LENSES

The patient should wear the disruptive prism lenses as well as red/green lenses. If the patient wears prescription lenses for acuity, then he or she should wear those glasses underneath.

SET-UP

Hang the ball so that it falls to the chest level of the patient. Place the chair four feet from, and facing, the ball. Direct the patient to sit in the chair. Adjust the lenses of the 20-degree adjustable prism into the base-up and base-down position, so that the thick part of the right lens is on the top of the frame and the thick part of the left lens is on the bottom of the frame. Place the red and green lenses underneath the 20-degree adjustable prism lenses. If the patient benefits from proprioceptive feedback (his or her muscular system directing the visual system) the patient may hold a pointer or chopstick in the dominant hand. Lastly, the trainer should place the bean bag toy, hat, or another light-weight object on top of the patient's head.

OBJECTIVE

Creating awareness of depth, and increasing eye movements to reorganize the patient's visual perceptual processing.

PROCEDURE

Part I—static: Ask the patient to look at the ball. Next, ask the patient how many balls he or she sees. When looking at the ball, the patient should actually see two balls, one red and the other green. Continue asking the patient to distinguish the differences between the two balls. The patient may describe differences in height (one ball is above the other) and depth (where one ball will appear closer to the patient than the other). If the patient is unaware of these differences, the trainer should wait a few minutes before verbally prompting the patient for those differences.

Part II—dynamic: Once the patient sees two balls, distinguishes their differences, and has no difficulty maintaining the two, the trainer can set the ball in motion. The ball should swing in a horizontal plane in front of the patient. Direct the patient to watch the two balls as they swing back and forth. If the patient has difficulty following the balls, direct the person to use the chopstick to follow the ball as it swings from side to side *or* to "hit the red ball!" or "hit the green ball!" with the chopstick. Encourage the patient to keep a straight and level head and to breathe in a relaxed manner when tracking the balls.

OBSERVATIONS

- Is the patient aware of two balls, or does he or she only see one?

- Does the patient distinguish the differences in color, height, and depth?

- Can the patient track the ball comfortably with his or her eyes, or does the patient require the use of the chopstick?

TIME
Spend approximately five minutes on this procedure.

RESULTS
This procedure has a dramatic effect on patients with these issues:

1. *Anxiety:* Leads to immediate relaxation.

2. *Tunnel vision:* Makes the room appear larger.

3. *Emotions:* Increases motivation due to release of tension.

VISUAL ISSUES AT DIFFERENT AGES AND STAGES

5 VISUAL DYSFUNCTION IN THE ACTION-ORIENTED CHILD

Childhood is an apprenticeship. In our earliest days as action-oriented infants and children, we have a very important job: to rehearse the interrelationship of mind, body, and world.

In order to move from that rehearsal to a flawless performance, we need to master two goals in our early years. The first goal is to orient ourselves to our space world. This allows us to create visual maps, ground our posture, and control our movements as we interact with the world. The second goal is to create a body schema—a knowledge of where "self" ends and the outside world begins. This allows us to transform sensory information quickly so we can answer the questions, "Where am I?" and "Where is it?"

If children master these two goals, they can maneuver their bodies easily. But if they hit a roadblock, symptoms can include anything from toe-walking to scoliosis to emotional and learning problems. When we approach these symptoms as clues to solutions rather than as unsolveable problems, we can understand them—and often, we can correct them. Here are some examples from my own practice.

Dan: toe-walking as a visual-mapping delay

As children move from crawling to walking, they often begin by toe-walking. The question most first-time parents ask when they see this is "Should I be alarmed?"

The renowned Mayo Clinic offers the mainstream medical consensus on this issue. According to them, toe–walking often is idiopathic—that is, "we don't know why it happens." The Mayo Clinic says many infants toe-walk to some degree through their toddler years. Most will outgrow it, the doctors at Mayo say, while others will continue to do it out of habit.

My concept of toe-walking is different. I believe it is a delay of visual mapping. Just like an adult trying to follow an inaccurate road map, a child who toe-walks has difficulty moving through his world.

When we walk normally, we step forward on our heels and land on our toes. But ask toe-walkers to walk on a flat surface, and they step forward on their toes and stay on their toes. This is because they need to attend to the floor's two-dimensional surface to guide them visually.

Toe-walking causes a child's center of gravity to move forward. To achieve postural stability in this awkward position and avoid falling down, the toe-walker needs to rush to get to a destination. It's interesting to observe seniors in their twilight years come full circle as they return to toe-walking and rush when they walk.

The question is: Should toe-walking be treated? The answer itself is quite controversial. Many doctors say no. Others recommend treatment, including stretching, casting, orthotics, or even surgery, for children who do not outgrow this behavior. The point of these medical therapies is to change structure in order to affect function.

But there doesn't need to be any controversy in cases where we can change function *without* changing structure. For example, consider what happens when you ask toe-walkers to walk slightly uphill. Their center of gravity moves back, their gaze moves up, and they walk in a normal heel-to-toe gait.

Now consider what happens when we apply base-down yoked prisms to toe-walking children. These prisms create an illusion, making a flat surface appear inclined. The eyes lead the mind, causing these children to believe they are walking uphill, and they respond with a normal heel-to-toe gait.

This is the approach I used with Dan, a ten-year-old who was being treated medically for toe-walking. His orthopedist started with a conservative treatment of stretching and braces. The doctor told Dan's mother that if the conservative approach failed, the next step would be to cut the tendons in his calves to stretch the muscles.

Two months into treatment, Dan's mother decided to get another opinion. She'd read an article about my approach and wanted to give it a try.

Dan arrived at my office wearing his braces. As he walked in, his head and shoulders were forward and down. My first thought was that he was living in a two-dimensional world and needed to look at the floor to guide his gait. But I held my comments until after Dan's examination.

The examination revealed that Dan's visual perceptual style was normally global—that is, involving ambient (peripheral) vision. However, in order to function, he was overcompensating and relying on his focal (central) vision, making him see the world in 2-D.

Dan's overcompensation showed in his visual performance. He had difficulty tracking, he had tunnel vision, and he had delays in mapping his body schema. His orientation issues also led to poor balance.

I explained to Dan's mother that his toe-walking was just one symptom of the steps he'd skipped in development. I also explained that his overcompensation would likely lead to behavioral issues in school, at play, and in social interactions. In addition, he would probably display anxiety or explosiveness at times, and he would finally shut down.

His mother said, "You got all this from an eye examination?" I replied, "The old Greeks had it right: Why blame the eyes when it's the brain that does the seeing?"

Dan, his mother, and I went into the therapy room. I asked Dan to walk across the room while looking at himself in the mirror on the opposite wall. Dan walked on his toes, looking at the floor. Then I asked Dan to take off his braces and repeat the procedure. Once again, he walked across the room on his toes.

At that point, I placed 20-diopter base-down prisms on Dan and said, "Let's repeat walking to the mirror." This time, Dan walked normally, heel-to-toe.

I then asked Dan to stand and said, "Let's play catch." I saw immediate apprehension on his face. When the ball came toward him, his head jerked back and his hand missed the ball. I had him sit down and again threw the ball at him. This time his head jerked back, but he caught the ball.

Next, I placed 2-diopter base-up yoked prisms on him. This time, Dan reached out and caught the ball, holding his head still. The final time I asked him to stand while wearing the prisms, and he caught the ball easily.

Like other toe-walkers, Dan functioned in a compressed, two-dimensional world. When I initially applied 20-diopter ambient base-down yoked prisms, this transformed his visual field into a wide-angle three-dimensional field, creating a conscious change in adaptation that he demonstrated by immediately walking normally. Because his perceptual style was ambient but he overcompensated by tunneling, I then switched to 2-diopter base-up ambient yoked prisms in order to transform his perception so he could capture depth with improved timing.

I've treated hundreds of children like Dan, with similar results. In my view, idiopathic toe-walking is not idiopathic and not "normal." It is a delay in the development of a child's self-organization of mind, body, and world, and failure to address it may affect the child's overall development.

In order to grasp this, a medical professional must look beyond the child's gait, or for that matter the function of his or her eyes. Understanding toe-walking means looking at the whole child and identifying the problems that child is solving through this behavior.

Nadine: postural warps and the role of the vestibulo-ocular reflex

In Chapter 1 I talked about the vestibulo-ocular reflex (VOR). This mechanism allows our gaze to remain stable when the head moves, letting us maintain balance and clear vision.

To understand this, think of a camera. How often have you taken a picture with an unsteady hand and discovered that your pictures came out blurry? The eye, like the camera, must be held steady by the "photographer" (in this case, the VOR) in order to produce a clear picture.

When the VOR isn't working correctly, people must find solutions in order to adapt to their world. And the solutions they find will depend a great deal on how severe their dysfunction is.

Nadine, a six-year-old girl whose parents brought her to my office as a last resort, had responded to her abnormal VOR with extreme solutions. Her current doctor had labeled her as having "cortical neural impairment," just one of the many diagnoses she'd received over her short lifetime.

Nadine's mother wheeled her into my office. She was nonverbal and kept her eyes narrowed most of the time, and her body was in an almost fetal position. An orthopedic physician had placed her in braces from knee to ankle that caused her to cry every time they were applied.

While Nadine was nonverbal, she did respond to speech. But neither conventional visual testing nor my Kaplan Nonverbal Battery (see Appendix II) was appropriate in her case. So I decided to try disruptive yoked prisms.

First, I had Nadine sit up in her carriage while watching a music video. She didn't respond even with 20-diopter (high-magnitude) base-down yoked prisms.

My next thought was to try something active rather than passive. So I asked Nadine's parents to remove her painful leg braces. Then I asked them to stand her up, with one parent supporting her on either side. Her body slumped, her head tilted down and right, and her legs bowed.

Next, I placed the 20-diopter base-down yoked prisms on Nadine and stood back to observe. It didn't take long before we saw a change. She started to roll her head around slowly, and I could see her eyes opening.

At this point, I asked her parents to keep supporting Nadine's body while walking with her. I expected her feet to drag across the floor. However, Nadine started to raise her legs as if she were walking up an incline. It was obvious she was responding to the transformation of her spatial world.

I was excited to see her responding, but she became visibly tired and we stopped and returned her to the carriage. Nadine's performance was encouraging, but her prognosis was still guarded. I explained to her parents that I needed more information before we could decide on a course of treatment.

I showed Nadine's parents how to apply the disruptive prisms in different directions and taught them a few visual motor procedures to use at home two or three times a day. Then I asked them to come back in a month.

On her return to the office, there wasn't a dry eye as Nadine—wearing the prism lenses and no braces—walked into the office on her own.

Liz: when poor visual orientation leads to problems in movement and learning

Liz was a four-year-old in private school when I first saw her. She had severe learning issues, and her teacher said that she would never be able to make normal academic progress. Liz's mother, who refused to give up on her, brought the girl to my office. Later, she sent me this letter about the effects of Liz's vision therapy.

> I found Dr. Kaplan through a friend who suggested my daughter might benefit from meeting him. After a full year on the waiting list, Liz finally had the chance to meet Dr. Kaplan. It was worth the wait although painful to think of the year that passed and how things might have been different for our family had we seen him sooner.
>
> Liz was a little over four years old when she had her initial appointment with Dr. Kaplan. While in a special needs preschool, receiving occupational, physical, and speech therapies, Liz had no specific diagnosis. The simplest way to describe her was to say something was "off." She was a very sickly child, in a pattern of almost one week sick, one week healthy. Her energy level was

poor and her disposition difficult. Cognitively she was inconsistent—age appropriate in some areas and behind in others. Physically she was uncoordinated, imbalanced and stressed by dynamic environments—she was unwilling/unable to throw, catch or hit a ball, would pedal a bike a few times and quit, and would trip, fall and run into things constantly. While socially she was outgoing, she was inappropriate—talking to teachers who were across the room as if they were standing next to her, going from classmate to classmate repeating the same thing to each, etc. Needless to say, a very adept child study team acknowledged her shortcomings and placed her in a special needs program. After her first year in the program, her case manager, appropriately or not, informed us that she expected Liz to be in a special education program for the foreseeable future.

In September, we saw Dr. Kaplan for the first time. Within the first two minutes of the exam, Dr. Kaplan asked Liz to stand on one foot. She attempted to do so as her face grimaced, her hands flailed, and quickly she had to put her foot down. Dr. Kaplan put glasses on her and asked her to try again. She stood like a statue and I was reduced to tears. The exam continued, converting me into a believer much more quickly than my skeptical husband. Trying to process the immediate and dramatic change in our daughter was challenging—but we saw the results firsthand. In fact, my husband went one step beyond and had Dr. Kaplan test him. My skeptical husband now wears the glasses, plays tennis at a higher level, and is able to read more than two pages of a book before falling asleep.

The changes in Liz are almost too far-reaching to list as we now can appreciate how challenging her world once was. Her digestive issues, her low energy levels, her difficult temperament, and her chronic health problems have all disappeared.

Never would I have imagined her visual function would be related to all of these seemingly tangential characteristics. Looking back, it all makes sense. When someone is tense as a result of their not feeling visually stable, their body is exhausted trying to compensate, thereby causing many physiological issues.

Cognitively, Liz has shown tremendous progress as well. She has quickly learned her letter sounds, can count and can reason—all contributing to her being placed in a mainstream preschool for a few days each week. She also has grown physically. She now initiates throwing and catching, and has even learned to write.

While it would be difficult for Liz to comprehend the reason for her glasses and her exercises, she knows how she feels. She never takes her glasses off and works hard at her exercises. She clearly feels better wearing her glasses. At her most recent IEP [individualized education program] meeting, one teacher described her as "the happiest child she had ever met." And she is right.

Liz's case wasn't an isolated incident. In fact, I've seen many children like her, so I knew what to look for.

The first clue to Liz's developmental delay came when she entered the room and walked across the floor to look at herself in the mirror. As I watched her, I saw that Liz's left shoulder was lower than her right and her left foot toed in. Normally, the shoulders should be even, and both feet should be slightly toed outward.

It is well established that our brain's right hemisphere controls the left half of our body, and maps the geography of our world. In Liz's case, this didn't happen correctly. So her mind's solution was to compress her attention to the right side of her body. The loss of the interaction between both sides of her body and the compression of her field of view increased the time it took for her mind, body and world to interact. The consequences of her adaptive solution included problems with posture, balance, and laterality (that is, knowing her left from her right).

At this point, I needed to determine whether Liz's symptoms were structural or functional. I assessed this through pre- and post-tests. First, I asked Liz to look at herself in a mirror and raise one foot. Developmentally, a child her age should be able to hold her balance through the count of ten. Liz was unable to raise and hold up her leg and fell to the side. Then I placed base-left yoked prisms on Liz and asked her to try again. She not only was able to raise her leg, but was able to sustain her balance. The base-left prisms gave her a greater awareness of the left side of her body.

With therapy, we were able to make the temporary changes created by the prism lenses permanent. Therapy allowed Liz's field of vision to expand outward so she could accept information outside the tunnel world she'd enclosed herself in. She was able to develop a more accurate body schema— the egocentric awareness of "where am I?"—which enabled her to identify the relative location and orientation of her body parts. She also developed the skills she needed in order to understand her relationship to places, objects, and events. And over time, she was able to develop a firm concept of left and right and to move easily in three-dimensional space.

As a result of these changes, Liz became a happier, more confident child. Her health improved dramatically, and so did her emotional stability. And she clearly proved her teacher wrong—demonstrating that when a professional says a child can't learn, it's time to get a second opinion.

Developing a learning style

As children begin to orient themselves to their world and develop a body schema, they also begin to exhibit their individual learning styles. Educational experts Rita Dunn and Shirley Griggs (2000) describe learning styles as the way an individual "begins to concentrate on processing, internalizing, and remembering new information and skills."

One category of learning styles is based on sensory preferences: visual, auditory, or tactile (touch). Each child develops a unique brain pathway preference for taking in and thinking about information. Early in life, it takes two or more sensory pathways to lock in received information—*see and hear, see and touch, hear and touch,* etc. Over time, children focus increasingly on one of these senses.

Another category of learning style exists *within* the visual system. In visual perception, information follows two different pathways from the eye to the brain's visual cortex: focal and ambient. People whose minds favor a focal path work in a predictably logical, orderly fashion and prefer process-driven environments. Those who favor an ambient path prefer more open-ended situations, moving from task to task.

For focal processors, eye movements are sequential, as are thought processes. In ambient processors, eye movements are more saccadic (jumpy) and their thoughts are global. These visual perceptual styles are often overlooked in both classrooms and the workplace. Yet in many cases, people's success in school or at work depends largely on whether their visual perceptual styles mesh well with real-life demands.

One child who illustrated this was Charlie, a second-grader with a command of spoken language far above his seven years. He had a great imagination, but he also exhibited delays in hand–eye coordination that caused him to have trouble with ball play, running, and handling tools. He was at the top of his class in math, and it came as a complete surprise to his parents when a teacher told them he had issues in reading.

My office was their first stop. I found that Charlie's eye health and sight were normal. However, I discovered that he had issues with eye tracking, posture, and visual attention. My examination also showed that he had a strong preference for the ambient pathway in visual processing.

The parents' second stop was at the office of a speech audiologist, who investigated his auditory processing. The audiologist told them that Charlie had phonic receptive issues. However, because he was so bright, his speech and language processing were above age level. The audiologist's advice was, "Don't worry about his reading—he'll catch up."

I was invited to meet with Charlie's teacher. Her suggestion was to take Charlie to a reading specialist. However, I had a different idea.

I told the teacher that I'd detected eye movement issues that would affect Charlie's ability to keep his place. I explained that reading, from a neurobiological behavior point of view, involves both "where" and "what." First, a child must find where the print is, and second, the child must comprehend what the print means.

I asked the teacher what method she was using to teach Charlie to read. She answered, "Phonics." I explained that, in addition to his vision issues, Charlie had issues with phonetic listening, and that this could be an additional cause of his reading delay. We compromised by implementing a look-see program. Because this approach matched Charlie's preferred learning style (ambient) rather than focusing on his weak areas, I knew it would be more effective for him than phonics.

In the meantime, Charlie participated in a visual therapy program. At the end of the program, Charlie's posture and attention were markedly improved. In fact, he even joined a soccer team. His teacher was happy with his progress in reading as well.

When Charlie entered third grade, the teacher's conference was quite different from the previous one. The new teacher had reviewed his individualized education program and told his parents that she was surprised to see that he had reading issues in the second grade. She said, "He's only in the third grade, and he's reading on a ninth-grade level."

Viewing vision as a system

Charlie, like many children with reading problems who come to my office, didn't simply need more practice in reading. Instead, he needed an educational approach that focused on his strengths—and he needed therapy to address not his eyes (which functioned normally), but the software of his visual system.

The visual system, as famed developmental expert Arnold Gesell (1950) wrote, "is more than a dioptric lens and a retinal film. It embraces enormous areas of the cerebrum; it is deeply involved in the autonomic nervous system; it is identified reflexively and directively with the skeletal musculature from head and hand to foot." This holistic nature of vision explains why visual deficits can affect everything from reading to walking to behavior.

Gesell (1950) also stated a crucial fact: that vision is "pervasively bound up with the past and present performances of the organism," because each stage in the integration of the visual system builds on previous stages. And it is these early stages of development—and the consequences of missing stages—that I'll discuss in the next chapter.

6

THE HIGH COST OF SKIPPING STEPS

In most cases, the patients I see in my office struggle to create their visual worlds because they have missed crucial steps in their early development. These missed milestones often translate into visual perceptual problems and developmental delays in areas ranging from postural control and movement to language, social, and cognitive skills.

To put these developmental delays into perspective, we need a blueprint that describes how development normally progresses. The famous developmental biologist Jean Piaget described these four stages of cognitive development:

- *Sensorimotor*—birth through 18 to 24 months: In this stage, children begin to understand the world by seeing, hearing, and interacting with it.

- *Preoperational*—toddlerhood (18 to 24 months) through early childhood (age 7): Here, children begin to exhibit pretend play but can't yet use concrete logic and have difficulty seeing other people's points of view.

- *Concrete operational*—age 7 to 12: At this point, children begin using logic but still cannot think abstractly. They can distinguish between other people's feelings and thoughts and their own.

- *Formal operational*—adolescence through adulthood: At this stage, people are capable of hypothetical and deductive reasoning.

One of my mentors, Arnold Gesell M.D., established his own model to describe the stages of growth. Gesell based his model on the premise that to know a child's behavior, one must know the child's visual system—and to know the visual system of a child, one must know the child. As Gesell (1950) understood, a child's behavior and his vision are inseparable.

Based on my own clinical experience and scientific studies, I have built on Gesell's foundational ideas. In my model, I view the human organism as a *spatial action system*. As I see it, there are crucial steps, such as releasing objects at nine months or crawling on all fours later in infancy. If these steps are missed, problems occur later in life.

These are the three major stages of perceptual development an individual passes through:

- *Stage 1:* The action-specific child (birth to 10 years).

- *Stage 2:* The adaptive adolescent (11 to 17 years).

- *Stage 3:* The thought-oriented adult (18 years and older).

Piaget's stages correspond to the development of intellect, thought, judgment, and knowledge. My own approach focuses on other important aspects of human development, including action, adaptation, and perception, and how these affect posture, attention, emotion, and behavior. Piaget's model is conscious; mine is preconscious.

Both Piaget's model and mine recognize that some children may pass through developmental stages at different ages than the expected times. Also, skipping steps may cause a child to show characteristics of multiple stages.

In my model, skipping stages invariably impacts both performance and perceptual adaptation. Missed milestones interfere with people's ability to reach their full intellectual potential and are the underlying cause of many emotional disorders.

Skipping steps results in compression or suppression of a person's world view and knowledge. The solutions that people find to cope with their developmental delays further reduce their knowledge and increase the time it takes to process input.

As a result, skipped steps can lead to physical problems as diverse as scoliosis (curvature of the spine) and strabismus (improper eye alignment). By identifying these missed steps and addressing them, vision therapy can powerfully address these problems, as the cases in this chapter show.

Michael: when missed steps lead to scoliosis

Scoliosis is a lateral curvature of the spine that exceeds ten degrees. Some cases of scoliosis stem from medical conditions such as cerebral palsy or spina bifida. However, most cases of scoliosis are considered idiopathic; that is, doctors believe they have no clear underlying cause.

What *is* clear, in my opinion, is that these idiopathic cases do not stem from structural issues. Orthopedic specialist J. Abbott Byrd III M.D. (1988) writes, "Abnormalities of disc, bone, muscle and collagen do not appear to be etiological factors, but rather reflect the effects on normal tissues." He adds, "It appears that a brain stem or equilibrium abnormality does exist in patients with idiopathic scoliosis." Similarly, Richard Herman M.D., medical and research director at Good Samaritan Hospital in Phoenix, Arizona (Herman *et al.* 1985), says experiments show that people with idiopathic scoliosis suffer from a disturbance in "visual spatial perception."

This disturbance appears to stem from a problem in the brain's magno (ambient) pathway, which I'll talk more about in Chapter 8. In scoliosis, there often is a flaw in the visual perceptual message because the magno system does not correctly interpret how upright the body is.

I see many adolescents with scoliosis who are referred to my office for learning or social issues rather than for scoliosis. In my experience, both these teens' spine curvature and their learning and social problems stem from skipped developmental steps, and we can address all of these issues by retraining the brain.

Michael, a 16-year-old, was a typical example. Although Michael had a high IQ, he was falling behind academically. His father, a local dentist, had heard that I was having success in treating issues related to academics.

Michael entered my office wearing a body brace, a non-surgical approach to idiopathic scoliosis. He told me that he loved playing tennis (although he had some issues at the net) but he wasn't too crazy about academics.

Michael's performance on the Visual Skills Test and Kaplan Star Test (see Appendix I) told me that he would have issues with eye movements, spatial organization, spatial orientation, and attention to task. Further testing confirmed this profile. He displayed saccadic (jumpy) eye movements, poor eye contact, and issues in keeping his place when he read—all symptoms associated with poor spatial organization. And in tasks requiring spatial orientation, it was obvious he had missed crucial developmental steps.

Children with problems like Michael's have two choices in coping with their problems: facing them (fight) or escaping them (flight). While other 16-year-olds with his brain power would work hard to do well academically, Michael chose avoidance. When he became stressed while reading, he'd simply turn his attention elsewhere. There was only one place where he was up for the challenge: on the tennis court.

I knew from experience that telling Michael that I could make him a better student wouldn't motivate him. So instead, I told him I could improve his net game.

With his parents watching, I threw a ball to Michael and he pulled it into his body. I asked him to sit, and threw the ball to him again. This time, he reached out a bit and caught it. However, his head jerked back.

I repeated this procedure with Michael wearing ambient yoked prisms. This time, he caught the ball with relaxed attention, both while sitting and while standing.

I spoke privately to his parents, who were quite excited to see how motivated he was after my demonstration. I told them that in my experience, visual processing issues like Michael's contribute to academic, social, and emotional delays. I also told them that I expected therapy to lead to improvements not just in these areas but also in his scoliosis as we enhanced his ability to process information.

Michael attacked the program with great enthusiasm and wore the lenses religiously. As a result, his academic abilities soared—and so did his net game in tennis.

At the end of the sixth week, Michael went back to the orthopedic surgeon who had been contemplating surgery. The doctor told his parents that he was amazed: Michael had gone from a 20-degree curvature to 12 degrees, and the doctor felt that surgery was no longer necessary.

Michael's story shows how missed steps affect not only learning and emotional stability but also posture. His visual processing deficits had forced him to focus too much attention on where he was in space, causing a postural warp.

Attention can be defined as "the information processing capacity of an individual." There is a limit to how much information a person can process, and the extra demand on Michael's attention reduced his capacity to attend to postural control. When therapy freed Michael to pay less attention to his position in space, the logical result occurred: his posture improved.

By the way, when Michael's father asked the surgeon what he felt caused the change in curvature, the doctor replied, "The plasticity of the spine." When Michael's father explained about his son's visual management program, the surgeon said it wouldn't have had any impact. Although I achieve similar results with other patients again and again, it's difficult to convince orthopedic doctors to look beyond braces and surgeries and consider addressing the brain's software instead.

When Michael first came to my office, his primary issues involved delays in orienting himself to his space world and to his own body's position. As a result, both his schoolwork and his posture had suffered. But Kelly, the patient I'll talk about next, had a very different set of problems due to missed developmental steps that prevented her from organizing her space world accurately.

Kelly: when missed steps lead to strabismus

In strabismus, the eyes fail to align with each other. Left untreated, strabismus can lead to amblyopia, or lazy eye, in which the brain ignores the input from one eye.

The general consensus of doctors is that while some cases of strabismus stem from neurological or muscular disorders, most cases are idiopathic. Typically, physicians focus on correcting visual acuity by patching one eye—or, if that doesn't work, by performing surgery to make some eye muscles stronger or weaker.

However, I approach strabismus in a very different way, by focusing on function rather than structure. Strabismus involves neural control, not muscle strength. (In fact, doctors admit that while the eyes may look straight after surgery, vision problems often remain.) Eye movements are a function of the ambient visual pathway, and therefore I direct my treatment toward neural reorganization in this pathway. The goal is a reprogramming of visual information processing, leading to a higher level of performance and behavioral adaptation.

Another way to explain my approach is that I view both strabismus and amblyopia as a question of *where* rather than a question of *what*. The *what* is the end product—a loss of acuity and binocularity. But the *where* is an issue involving not only the eyes but the individual as a whole, due to skipped steps in development, and that is what I treat.

While the structural model focuses on straight eyes and (sometimes) good acuity, my goal is improved visual organization that will lead to better performance and behavior. In my approach, acuity improves as part of the outcome.

How effective is this approach? Rather than describing the results myself, I'll let Kelly—one of my patients, who also was a member of my staff for several years—describe them in her own words.

> I remember the first time someone called me "cross-eyed." It was in fourth grade during recess after a long morning of English and social studies. At my young age, I interpreted being "cross-eyed" as having a learning issue

and cried to my mom when I got home. She assured me that my eyes were perfectly fine.

Then, a few years later, I was at my general practitioner's office when he said to my mom, "Does Kelly's eye turn in?" As he checked by shining a light into both of my eyes, he attributed the appearance of an eye turn to facial asymmetry.

When I got to optometry school, they defined this "cross-eye" as esotropia, a condition where there is a misalignment between the two eyes. Most often, one eye is looking straight ahead and the other has an inward deviation.

Esotropia has been a part of my life since a young age. As a self-conscious teenager, I picked up that my eye would turn in when I was tired and had been at school all day. All of my sisters have the same thing (it was sort of the family joke that we could tell who was the most tired by whose eye was turned in the most), so I just wrote it off as genetic and something I'd have to deal with. High school was a breeze academic-wise—I was in the top ten of my class, while balancing a job, clubs, and sports. College came, and although the course load was difficult, I was again able to balance a job, holding executive positions in clubs, having a social life, and excelling in my academics.

This time, however, my success came at a cost: I was constantly stressed. Not only in my everyday life, but in my body. My shoulders were tense, and I often felt myself tightening up my jaw as I studied. I found that I was no longer able to keep my concentration well, having to re-read things three or more times as opposed to my normal one to two times in high school. Due to this excessive reading, I needed to take more breaks (which was quite frustrating as I never had an issue before sitting down and studying for hours on end).

On top of the stress, I noticed that I was getting fatigued more often. I would be exhausted after just a two-hour lecture! Even my eyes seemed "tired"—almost like they didn't want to, or couldn't, focus on all the near work I was doing. The only way I found to deal with all of these things was going to the gym. I found myself going to the gym twice a day because it was the only way I could figure out how to relax my body and clear my mind.

The middle of my sophomore year of college, I began working for Dr. Kaplan. The first thing he said to me when he met me was, "You have visual problems." I responded by saying, "I know, I wear glasses." He smirked and said to me lightly, "You have more problems than that."

As taken aback as I was, I knew he was right. Being the person that I am, I just always fought through my fatigue, stress, and eye strain. I figured it was the price I had to pay to be successful. Luckily, I stumbled upon the right guy to show me that life doesn't have to be that hard.

He prescribed me a pair of glasses and like magic, all of my issues started to disappear. I began doing vision therapy alongside of wearing these glasses to rewire and solidify new visual habits to help me use my eyes in a more efficient manner. Through this training, I realized my visual system was expending so much energy that it was taking away from other aspects that I needed to function. My stress, fatigue, and lack of comprehension were all a result of my visual adaptations in order to continue my level of success.

How you feel when you put prisms on is sort of unexplainable. It is sort of something you can't believe until you try it yourself. The effects are so immediate that it is almost too good to be true. When I would wear the glasses, I found that both my body and my eyes were relaxed. There was no longer that struggle to keep focus on the page and I sure didn't have a tense back!

When it came to comprehension, it'd be safe to say that it increased at least ten-fold. I didn't have to re-read as much and the concepts seemed to just come together. I guess you can say that my thinking and understanding became clearer and smoother; that is, I no longer had to force the connections to be made.

Now that I am in graduate school, I am doing more close work than ever. The stress of all the assessments and studying has sometimes got me in a frenzy, but my lenses have kept my body and eyes relaxed—allowing me to be more successful than ever before.

When missed steps translate into symptoms like Michael's or Kelly's, doctors typically look at each individual symptom rather than seeing the whole picture. That's why they treat scoliosis with braces and surgery, and why they treat strabismus with eye patches and surgery.

But missed steps don't just affect the back or the eye. They affect every aspect of a person's life, and individual symptoms usually reflect a larger breakdown in orientation and organization. Address this breakdown, and you will see changes not just in one or two symptoms but in many areas of life. Katherine, the next patient I talk about, is a good example.

Katherine: when missed steps lead to double vision

At the age of 15, Katherine was dragged to my office by her mother. Her behavior made it clear that she wanted to be anywhere but visiting me.

Katherine was fighting to get an education and to succeed as an athlete. But her skipped developmental steps, and the solutions she'd found to deal with them, left her struggling in both areas.

Katherine's exam indicated that she had intermittent double vision both at a distance and at near point. She could maintain fusion with large print, but only for short periods of time. Her visual perception, both far and near, showed a total lack of constancy. She had tunnel vision, needing to use a one-eyed "cyclops" approach to maintain control. The pattern on her Kaplan Star Test showed that her vision was compressed in the frontal plane; she preferred near to far space in the sagittal plane. Her star pattern was unorganized and indicated a fast alternating of binocular fields.

Katherine's profile indicated performance delays, balance issues, orientation problems, and organizational issues involving breathing and thinking. I correctly predicted that she would be a slow, word-by-word reader and would experience fatigue and headaches when she read. I also predicted that she would have many fears and anxieties.

My measurements confirmed that Katherine had double vision, leading her to suppress the input from one eye in order to see a single image. Although her eye movements appeared straight, her ocular alignment was highly tunneled. Katherine was able to track objects when they moved in a two-dimensional plane (*version* movement), but she was unable to turn her eyes inward or outward to track them (*vergence* movement).

When I asked Katherine to perform tasks that illustrated her visual problems, she was highly defensive. Despite her mother's wishes, she refused treatment.

Two years later, Katherine was back. This time, her vision problems were even worse. I learned that she was a coxswain on a boat and had caused it to crash. Yet despite this concrete evidence of her visual deficits, she still resisted the idea of treatment. I asked her, "Are you here because you want help, or because your mother insisted that you come?" She said, "Because my mother wanted me to come."

So I told her how I saw her future without therapy. Her issues would continue to accelerate, I said, and she probably would never finish college.

Katherine left the examination room, went to the bathroom, and became quite upset. But later she changed her mind and agreed to enter therapy. Here's how she described the results, in an interview with our staff.

. . . .

What visual, behavioral, and emotional systems were you experiencing before meeting with Dr. Kaplan?
I frequently would see double while I was reading or sitting in class. I also would have headaches after reading for long periods of time. I found myself re-reading the words on the page over and over again because I wouldn't comprehend what I had just read. I also was extremely tense and my shoulders always had giant knots in them that would never release.

I had a very difficult time relaxing and de-stressing. Many times my friends would tease me about being so clumsy and how I always managed to get hurt in seemingly ridiculous ways.

Did you initially think that any of your symptoms were unrelated to vision and later discover a connection?

I had no idea that my tension and clumsiness were related to my eyes. I sort of figured that they were two things I couldn't control and that I would just live with them for the rest of my life.

What changes did you notice during your first exam with Dr. Kaplan?

I noticed that as he would have me try different glasses, it became easier to read and to do the tasks he was asking of me. I felt that there was less strain behind my eyes and that I wasn't working as hard to concentrate.

If you can think back to the day of your visit and recall the thoughts going through your head, how did you feel once the exam was over?

I was overwhelmed with several different emotions. I was primarily shocked that someone who knew nothing about me could tell me so many details about myself, including things I had never even really acknowledged. I also was pretty upset, because although I had always done well in school and was convinced I was going to be successful in life, in one session I was told that if I continued down my same path, I was going to end up as a jobless college dropout. I was horrified. Or terrified, I'm not sure. But after a lot of tears, I realized that the visual management program might actually help and that Dr. Kaplan could be right. I accepted the challenge and started the program.

What changes did you see once you were in your glasses?

I found it a lot easier to read and did not have to force myself to concentrate. I could read for longer, and read smaller print, without having even the slightest headache. I could understand what I was reading the first time around, and so ultimately, I was able to read faster.

How long were you in a visual management program?

I was in the program for just about two years, from the fall of 2005 through the summer of 2007.

Were you prescribed lenses for full time, indoors, or near point? Were you comfortable wearing them some, most, or all of the time?

I initially was prescribed prisms for full-time use. I felt constantly dizzy and as if there were halos surrounding every bright light I saw, which was really scary during rush-hour traffic. They took me a while to get used to, but eventually I didn't even notice they were there.

After the full-time lenses, I had two separate pairs. I had one pair that was strictly for reading and near point, and I had another pair of sunglasses that I wore while I did crew. As the person in charge of steering the boat, I would often swerve and get scared that I was going to crash, even if I wasn't. The reading glasses were a little more constant and so they were easier to get used to than the sunglasses, but ultimately they both became a part of my daily routine and I felt no discomfort wearing them.

How are you doing now?

There are still a few, very rare times when I will see double, but it's usually only when I am really exhausted. It sort of seems like it's my body's way of telling me to get sleep. Other than the occasional double vision, I have found that reading is much easier and that I can remember what I read. I do find that I get distracted when I read, but by eliminating all distractions such as the television, music, or other people, I can really focus on what I am reading.

· ·

In order for Katherine's system to reorient and reorganize, I needed to empower her to open up and break out from her compressed view of her world. Her visual management program included lenses for indoor activity (low-plus and ambient yoked prisms) and perceptual activities with disruptive high-magnitude yoked prisms to create awareness of self (body) and stimulate her to perceive space outside her tunnel vision.

As Katherine's vision improved, so did her academic performance and her athleticism. She went from clumsy to graceful—and she succeeded in high school and, later, in college.

Katherine is living proof of Gesell's statement that a child isn't born with a visual world but must create it. Human vision is inherently *active* and *acted upon* by the environment.

Perception is a continuously emerging and ever-changing process, and adaptation is crucial for learning and emotional growth. When a person skips developmental steps, the process of adaptation fails and visual performance suffers. As a result, the world becomes chaotic and confusing.

If we address these missing steps, the child's visual world will become whole—and so will the child. But if we do not address them, the child's problems will persist and even worsen in adulthood.

Moving from action-specific child to adaptive adolescent: the changing role of the VOR

When action-specific children negotiate the early steps of development successfully, they enter what I call "adaptive adolescence." This is a transitional stage in which a child's preconscious mind moves from orienting the child in space to focusing his or her attention on the outside world. In the stage of adaptive adolescence, the child is capable of synthesizing cognitive, emotional, and environmental influences and experiences to create new knowledge, skills, values, and world views.

My guess is that at this point there is a shift in attention in the vestibulo-ocular reflex (VOR). Early in life, children's attention is led by their vestibulo system and supported by vision. By the time they reach the stage of adaptive adolescence, they are easily able to orient themselves to space. At this time, the visual aspect of the VOR takes the lead in directing attention, supported by the vestibular system.

The progression from childhood to adolescence follows the continuum of stages described by educational theorist David Kolb (1984). According to Kolb, learners perceive and process information in this continuum:

1. *Concrete experience:* Being involved in a new experience.

2. *Reflective observation:* Watching others or developing observations about one's own experience.

3. *Abstract conceptualization:* Creating theories to explain observations.

4. *Active experimentation:* Using theories to solve problems or make decisions.

The action-specific child exhibits the first two stages of this continuum, while the adaptive adolescent masters stages 3 and 4.

7 VISION DYSFUNCTION IN THE THOUGHT-ORIENTED ADULT

Children are action-oriented. They touch, they taste, they climb, and they jump. But when we reach adulthood, our actions are driven more by thought and less by action.

To function effectively as thinking adults, we need to make sense of the input we receive from our senses—especially our sense of vision. However, our ability to receive information far exceeds our capacity to understand it. To handle this overload, we need to filter out most of the data we receive and focus on what is important.

Adults who have skipped steps in development are unable to filter out unnecessary information. As a result, they need to use excessive amounts of body activity and memory to control the sensory information their brains receive. Mark, a professional who asked for my help, is a good example.

Mark: the disorganized banker

When Mark came for his appointment, I asked, "What is your issue?" He replied, "Visually organizing my office." I said, "Can you be a little more specific?" He told me that every time he accepted a higher-level promotion, he got a new office. His search for books, papers, or even pens and pencils created a great deal of visual stress. To compensate, he spent many hours a day memorizing where books and papers were placed so he could respond quickly just to keep up.

In a normal, ordered visual processing system, the mind and body can work together to unconsciously organize spatial and biological patterns. As a result, we can quickly filter out clutter and decrease unnecessary eye and body movements, optimizing our ability to organize and orient ourselves in space.

In Mark's case, however, his slow visual processing led to stress and chaos. Fortunately, he was smart enough to realize that this would only intensify as he climbed the corporate ladder, and he eagerly agreed to therapy. I designed a program of disruption and reintegration that made him consciously aware of his visual processes. As a result, he is now able to visualize his environment and solve problems in an appropriate period of time.

Like Mark, many adults have extreme difficulty organizing or orienting themselves in space. Often, this happens because the eyes are "taking turns" instead of working together—a problem called *binocular rivalry*. The faster a person needs to alternate between the two eyes, the more energy is required, and the more stressful it is for the person to process visual information. This was a severe problem for Andrew, whose visual processing impairment led to suicidal depression.

Andrew: the depressed patient with binocular rivalry

In day-to-day life, people with normal binocular vision generally don't experience binocular rivalry (although they may experience suppression in some visual regions). That's because even though the two eyes are seeing slightly different pictures, the brain can combine them to create a single image.

People with visual deficits, however, often experience binocular rivalry—a problem that's both unsettling and potentially dangerous. The solution is to plan a vision therapy program that addresses their intraocular conflicts.

"Ambiguous perception" and visual behavior

You're probably familiar with this famous optical illusion, called the Rubin Illusion, which looks like a vase if you perceive it in one way, and like two faces if you perceive it in another way. As the eye focuses alternately on figure and then on ground, you will see the two images alternate. You can probably feel your eye muscles move when you alternate between the two images.

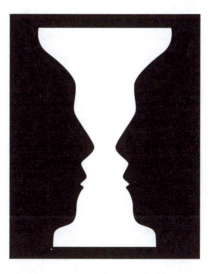

This is an example of what we call *ambiguous perception*. It's caused by eye movements that are out-of-sync in their search for information in the environment. This results in binocular rivalry that affects the stability of retinal images. This is entertaining when you are viewing an optical illusion, but crippling when you see your world this way.

Ambiguous perception stems from processing glitches in the dorsal and ventral pathways that provide information to the visual cortex of the brain. The ventral pathways carry information that allows us to identify objects ("What is it?"), and the excessive eye movements caused by the loss of binocular integration can result in low-power astigmatism and blurry images, making the "What is it?" question harder to answer. The dorsal pathway carries information related to spatial mapping ("Where is it?"), and spatial mapping disorders due to binocular rivalry lead to suppression and compression of a person's vision.

. . . .

Andrew, a 35-year-old patient of mine, illustrated how effective a program to address binocular rivalry can be. Andrew was severely affected by this problem. He was taking medication for depression, and his partner told me that Andrew was having suicidal thoughts.

Andrew had 20/20 vision, and his eyes were free of pathology. However, his binocular eye tracking was chaotic. He exhibited out-of-sync eye movements, and his head and body movements were uncontrolled. My testing revealed patterns reflecting a similar pattern of chaotic self-organization, revealing that he moved in and out of diplopia (double vision), suppression, and disorganization.

I could tell that evaluating Andrew in an orderly way would be a waste of time. Instead, I tried a unique procedure that involved creating vertical diplopia (double vision) in order to break up his binocular rivalry. I placed 20-diopter prisms on him, one base-up and the other base-down, with red/green filters. Then I swung a ball from side to side in front of him. In general, this procedure should stop the rivalry immediately, because each eye should see a separate colored ball—one red and one green. As a result, they should no longer be competing to see a single image.

Andrew initially saw one ball. Then I guided him to make his mind aware that he was viewing two vertically separate balls, and his body relaxed immediately. He said, "It's just like taking a tranquilizer." The procedure broke Andrew's suppression and allowed him to attend to both figures simultaneously (binocular vision) without rivalry. When he accomplished this goal, he achieved freedom of movement in tracking and no longer had a need for suppression.

By the end of the session, I knew we could help Andrew. And indeed, following therapy, his vision became stable and his depression diminished.

Like Andrew, many of my patients with ambiguous visual perception receive a label of mental illness and a prescription for medication. What they need, however, is for someone to address their core problem: their visual impairments.

These impairments often become more debilitating as people become adults. Adult life is complex and challenging, and when you add in visual impairments, every day can be a struggle. One of my patients, a 40-year-old architect, is a good example.

Tom: the architect who couldn't read blueprints

Tom was in deep trouble at his job because he was technically efficient but biologically unprepared for the spatial organization demands of working on huge blueprints. This task requires an intact binocular visual system with proficient saccadic eye movements that allow a person to keep a large span of space stabilized on the retina (the "film" of the eye).

Tom had skipped steps in his visual development and as a result suffered from binocular rivalry, leading him to alternately suppress the input from his right or left eye. Initially, he was able to do his job with some effort. Over time, however, it took him longer and longer to complete his work. He developed crippling headaches, became less resilient, and finally developed depression.

Tom eventually made an appointment with Dr. Frederic Flach, a psychiatrist with whom I had a professional relationship for many years. Fred told Tom that his visual perceptual disorder might play a major role in his depression, and he referred Tom to my office for a consultation.

Tom told me, "When I'm working on an easel, if I cover point A with a pencil, I can see Point B." Because he alternated between his eyes, he saw his world as linear (left or right) rather than as unified fields (left and right overlapping). In an attempt to solve his problem, he first tried speeding up switching from one field to the other, which required a large expenditure of energy. It didn't work, because humans have a finite supply of energy, and alternation leads to errors. Two other solutions remained: compressing or suppressing his visual field of view. When he did either one, Tom found himself in a visual tunnel.

I put a treatment plan in place to make Tom consciously aware of his alternating suppression while his eyes were tracking. As a result, his system relaxed, and the fight between his right and left visual field processing ended. This took the stress out of his eyes, jaw, and neck, which had all been spasming as his mind tried to control his gaze.

With his attention relaxed, Tom was able to stabilize and unify his peripheral visual fields. His work improved, he found socializing much easier, and his self-image rose. Fred and I were happy to hear Tom tell us after a few months that he felt strong enough to terminate treatment.

Many adults with binocular rivalry or other visual perceptual problems suffer greatly, just as Mark, Andrew, and Tom did. Without therapy, these people's lives would be a constant struggle for survival—and many of them would lose this struggle. Based on my own professional experience, I suspect that thousands of people with visual perceptual problems wind up in institutions or even commit suicide because the pain of living with their problem is just too great.

However, some people are able to "get by" or even do well despite visual perceptual problems. Generally, there are two factors that explain why they succeed while other individuals struggle. These factors are *perceptual preference* and *resilience*.

The influence of perceptual preference

Each person's brain has a preference as to how it processes information As I evaluate my patients, I can observe two types of thinkers: *spatial thinkers* and *logical thinkers*.

Temple Grandin, probably the most famous individual with autism, is a spatial thinker who describes her way of processing as "thinking in pictures." She views words as a second language. Logical thinkers, on the other hand, think in words.

Spatial thinkers face a number of challenges when it comes to verbal expression. Academia favors logical thinkers, and when it comes to writing, logical thinkers have a distinct advantage over spatial thinkers in putting their words on the page. Spatial thinkers, on the other hand, are likely to have an advantage in creative fields such as art and design.

(As a spatial thinker myself, I find it easier to interact physically with my patients than to communicate with them verbally. In these pages, I've described my pre- and post-testing methods—for instance, having patients balance on one foot or catch a ball. My patients and their caregivers usually leave my office with a better understanding of my treatment management program, but they sometimes find it difficult to explain to spouses or friends—possibly because I'm better at "showing" than at "saying.")

People who have skipped too many steps have difficulty even if the demands of their lives mesh well with their particular visual preference, whether spatial or logical. But many unfortunate people experience a "double whammy"—first, because they have visual impairments, and second, because they choose careers and lifestyles that don't mesh well with their perceptual preference.

For example, I once administered a screening profile to six medical school students as part of a class I was teaching. One student's profile indicated that he was a spatial thinker with visual organization issues that would interfere with reading comprehension.

I told the student that his profile indicated reading issues. He told me that reading was not an issue. When I asked why, he replied, "I don't read." His adaptation was to give up visual processing for auditory processing (for instance, using a computer program that translated text into speech). This solution was working for him temporarily, but I knew he would experience increasing stress and possibly a breakdown as the pressures of medical school increased.

A similar case involved Henry, the 48-year-old father of a patient of mine who was diagnosed with learning issues. Henry's son was responding well to therapy, and Henry wanted to meet with me to tell me how pleased he was with his son's progress. However, as it turned out, he also wanted to talk about himself.

Henry told me that reading was very difficult for him. He couldn't read for any significant period of time without experiencing fatigue, headache, and dizziness.

My evaluation revealed that Henry was a spatial thinker whose gaze control was impaired and unstable. I prescribed plus lenses with yoked base-up prisms. Two weeks later, he called and said, "Where were you when I needed you?" He explained that decades earlier, he'd dropped out in his third year of medical school because of the stress his reading issues caused. Now, at 48, he was finding reading comfortable and pleasurable.

Jill, another medical school student, eventually wound up in my office after suffering a nervous breakdown. The pressure of her visual impairments, combined with a perceptual preference that made her studies excruciatingly difficult, had caused her to crack. She was a spatial thinker who fought her stress until she collapsed and wound up in the hospital.

I put Jill in a visual therapy program. One month into therapy, I decided to use a disruptive procedure. As she walked with disruptive base-down yoked prisms, she turned to me and said, "I am alive again." It was a bit scary for me, but I knew we'd had a breakthrough.

The influence of resilience

To some degree, we all have visual deficits. In deciding whether these deficits require intervention, the question a clinician needs to ask is: Does an individual have enough resilience to thrive in spite of his or her visual deficits? And as it turns out, many people do.

Years ago, I was involved in a double-blind study involving psychiatric patients at the Westchester Medical Center. The results showed that patients differed significantly from a control group on both conventional and novel visual assessments. These findings support the notion that visual perceptual disorders may be associated with, and may even cause, disability in some psychiatric patients. Interestingly, however, 20 percent of the staff members in the control group had similar visual perceptual problems. This finding implies that some of the staff members had enough resilience to keep their symptoms from becoming clinical.

To explain how important resilience is, I like to use the analogy of golf. In golf the cry, "Fore!" is one of the most stressful sounds you can hear. Basically, it signals danger and tells you to search rapidly for an errant ball that may cause harm. For most golfers, the sound of "Fore!" results in a moment of heightened awareness. But for some people, the stress caused by this sound can be immobilizing and even terrifying.

Now, imagine that due to visual deficits, your daily interaction with your environment is similar to constantly hearing a cry of "Fore." If your resilience is high, and you can mask your responses or quickly recover, you may experience few problems. Like the staff at the Westchester Medical Center, you may be able to cope well enough to get by or even do well. If your resistance is low, however, then work, school, and/or relationships can rapidly become overwhelming. You're likely to develop physical and emotional symptoms, and you could be labeled as learning disabled, anxious, depressed, emotionally disturbed, or even autistic.

In the following chapters, you will read the stories of individuals whose resilience was insufficient for them to cope with their visual impairments. As a result, these people suffered from a wide range of physical, emotional, and cognitive problems. Fortunately, all of them found relief through visual management therapy.

FOUR ASPECTS OF VISUAL DYSFUNCTION

Anxiety

Reduced empathy

Issues with consciousness and memory

Motion sickness

8 VISUAL PERCEPTUAL IMPAIRMENT AND ANXIETY

Sometimes in life, we're fully aware of our feelings—for instance, when we're amused by a joke or upset over a flat tire. But other times, our emotional experiences are so intense that they're literally hidden from our awareness. In dangerous situations powerful emotions like fear can overwhelm us, so our evolutionary wiring favors subconscious, emotional control over conscious, cognitive control.

Neuroscientist Joseph LeDoux (1998) notes, "If you take away the conscious subjective register of fear, you are left with the behavioral and physiological responses. The unconscious characteristics are bodily changes, expressive movements, physiologic processes, and motor phenomena."

Visual problems make the world a more threatening place, harder to navigate and more difficult to understand. This results in increased fear, but people with visual problems don't always register this fear on a conscious level. Instead, their visual problems may translate into tenseness, dizziness, rapid heart rate, sweating, and even panic attacks. Symptoms like these are what led Mason, a 60-year-old with visual processing problems, to my office.

Mason: the judge who couldn't cross the bridge

Mason, a court judge, planned to arrive at my office for an evaluation at 10:30 on a Friday morning. But at 10:15 he called and said, "I'm sorry—I can't do it."

Mason didn't cancel his appointment because he'd caught the flu, or because a trial ran late. He cancelled because he was terrified.

When he called us, Mason was on the other side of the Tappan Zee Bridge near my clinic. Overwhelmed by anxiety about driving across the bridge, he told us he'd need to reschedule for another day so his law clerk could do the driving.

Mason was embarrassed and apologetic, but my staff and I understood his predicament completely. Many people with visual perceptual impairments panic at the idea of crossing a bridge or driving down a freeway. Moreover, Mason's cancellation was the first important clue I obtained about his vision problems.

With the help of his clerk, Mason arrived at our office a few weeks later. When I evaluated him, I wasn't surprised at the results. The judge had severely impaired depth perception, and as a result, he viewed his world as if looking through a tunnel.

In reality, Mason's initial plan to cross the Tappan Zee on his own—although it failed—was a sign of great courage. To understand why, picture yourself driving on a seven-lane, three-mile-long bridge while you're looking through two cardboard toilet paper rolls. You can't see the cars on either side of you. You can't tell where the drivers behind you are going. You're not even sure where your own body is. And you're terrified because it's impossible to tell how close the traffic is to you and how fast it's moving.

For Mason, challenges like this were part of everyday life—not just on the road, but everywhere. In a courtroom setting or an office, where events often happened slowly and predictably, he could relax much of the time. But at a crowded ballpark, on a freeway, or crossing a busy street, his tunnel vision made it impossible for him to accurately see the movement around him. As a result, his anxiety left him light-headed, dizzy, or even paralyzed with fear.

. . . .

What's it like to have tunnel vision?

Researcher Hubert Dolezal (1982) once conducted a study in which he viewed his world through tubes that were similar to binoculars without lenses. He described the immediate perceptual changes that occurred:

- He had trouble keeping objects in his field of view, which made coordinated eye–hand pursuits (such as closing a door) difficult.

- He was surprised when objects or people entered his field of view.

- His perception of events was impaired. For instance, he couldn't follow the action in a movie until he moved far away from the screen.

- He found himself making small, rapid, involuntary head movements in an attempt to obtain more visual information.

Dolezal's reactions are uncannily similar to what my patients with tunnel vision describe. The difference is that for these patients, tunnel vision isn't an experiment. If they don't get help, it's a life sentence.

. . . .

For years, Mason had felt embarrassed and ashamed about the anxiety that was associated with his visual stress, seeing this problem as a sign of weakness or cowardice. As a judge who needed to be logical and organized, he also worried about the effects that his "mental" problems might be having on his work.

And in fact, Mason *did* have mental problems—but in his case, they were actually solutions.

Mentally, Mason couldn't process the input he received from his eyes. This made it dangerous for him to put himself in situations where he might get injured: in a crowd, on a bustling sidewalk, or driving on the Tappan Zee. So Mason's brain "solved" the problem by making him feel anxious each time he approached these situations.

Mason wasn't consciously aware that his anxiety stemmed from the dysfunctional way he perceived depth. And that's not surprising, because brain research has shown that our emotions are controlled from unconscious, "bottom-up" feelings and not from "top-down" conscious thought.

Like most of my patients, Mason paid attention to his conscious ability to see. What he wasn't aware of, however, was what happened *after* he saw. But Mason's issues weren't related to his visual hardware (although he did need reading glasses). Instead, Mason's issues stemmed from faulty software. His eyes were sending accurate data, but his brain couldn't use that information correctly. So he couldn't orient himself, and he couldn't organize where objects were in relation to each other or to him. As a result, he felt great anxiety—but he wasn't aware of the reason for his feelings.

The solution to Mason's problem wasn't to treat him with anti-anxiety medications, something his other doctors had recommended. Instead, the solution was to correct his visual problem by retraining his visual system. So that is what we did. And amazingly, only three months into his visual management program, Mason was able to drive to his appointments without experiencing anxiety or dizziness.

Toward the end of his therapy, Mason shared a story with me. He told me that when he'd presided over trials in the past, the lawyers would often move around quickly while speaking, and he'd have trouble following their arguments because it took all of his energy to track their movements. "Now I'm much better able to focus on what I hear," he told me. "As a result, I'm much more confident in my decisions."

Vision and "high anxiety"

Our visual system both receives and acts on information from our environment. And our responses to incoming information are clearly reflected in our performance.

For my patients, a common response to demands from the environment is anxiety. Anxiety, of course, is one of our most basic human emotions. Simply put, it's our response to a threat, whether real or imaginary. It's the "fight or flight" response that makes us want to either run away or go on the attack.

In Mason's case, what I recognized was a classic flight response. Every time he was trapped in a crowd or maneuvering through traffic, his brain told him to escape or avoid the situation. When this happened over and over, it took an enormous toll on him psychologically.

To understand why Mason's vision problems led to chronic anxiety even though he had perfect focal vision, think of his visual cortex as a factory with two kinds of workers: P cells (parvo) and M cells (magno). Each of these two sets of workers has its own special job. The P cells gather messages from the cone cells of the retina and use them to provide data about detail and color: "It's a red apple sitting on a blue plate that has a little chip on the rim." The M cells, on the other hand, pick up information from the rod cells, which are devoid of color but sensitive to motion over a wide area. They tell us things like "The dog is running toward me" or "The driver behind me is getting too close to my bumper."

Mason's P cells did their job just fine. In the courtroom, he could easily identify the face of a defendant or the stripes on the prosecuting attorney's tie. But the disconnect involving his M cells meant that he couldn't perceive motion quickly and efficiently—and that left him in a constant state of tension that escalated to panic in traffic or crowds.

Mason's body responded to his visual problems on an unconscious level, leading to non-specific symptoms ranging from panic to heart palpitations to avoidance of freeways. As his example shows, anxiety caused by visual perceptual problems can manifest itself in three ways:

- *In mental responses:* For instance, through emotional reactions, nervousness, panic, and distorted thinking.

- *In biological responses:* For example, through dizziness, sweating, blurred vision, palpitations, chest pain, and rapid breathing.

- *In behavior:* For instance, through pacing, tapping, jaw clenching, and avoidance of settings that bring on anxiety.

Now let's look at what happened to Mason as he approached the Tappan Zee Bridge.

First, Mason's brain sent a message to the sympathetic branch of his autonomic nervous system. In response, his nervous system went into "fight or flight" mode, releasing energy and priming his body for action.

At this point Mason's sympathetic nervous system reacted in an all-or-none manner. (As I like to say, "Fear is specific, but anxiety is global.") Symptoms occurred simultaneously throughout his body. Consciously, he may have only realized that he was sweating or trembling. But in reality, his entire body was reacting. He was breathing quickly and shallowly, he was clenching his jaw, his heart was beating fast, and his mind was racing.

Once Mason's symptoms started, they continued and even worsened for a long time. Normally in an anxiety reaction, the parasympathetic system (which generally opposes the sympathetic system) will fairly quickly return the body to a homeostatic state—that is, the balanced state of relaxation and tension that the body considers normal. But in chronic anxiety, sympathetic activity proceeds without any hindrance from the parasympathetic system. As a result, Mason's body continued to release chemicals that made him feel anxious well after the perceived threat was gone.

In his anxious state, Mason experienced respiratory symptoms. His rapid, shallow breathing led to breathlessness which, in turn, led to feeling choked or smothered or feeling pain or tightness in his chest. Hyperventilation reduced the blood supply to his brain, resulting in dizziness, blurred vision, confusion, feelings of unreality, and hot flashes.

Anxiety can also affect the eyes, causing a person's pupils to enlarge. Eye movements may become excessive, and the person's blink rate may increase. In addition, anxious people often change their posture and gait—for instance, tilting their shoulders forward and up, tilting their head or full body, or toe-walking. And finally, chronic or frequent bouts of anxiety may dramatically affect behavior, leading to verbal or physical aggression or efforts to escape.

In extreme cases, a person with visual perceptual problems may mentally suppress these responses to stress in order to protect the body from additional harm. However, as I'll explain in the next section, this suppression can cause its own damage.

The three stages of adaptation to stress

Hans Selye, a famous researcher and endocrinologist, spent much of his life studying the stress response. One of Selye's most important concepts is that if you experience stress responses over and over, you will adapt in three phases:

- *An alarm reaction:* This is your initial "fight or flight" response. Here, your body releases the stress hormones cortisol, adrenaline, and noradrenaline to give your body a quick shot of energy.

- *A stage of resistance:* At this point, your body attempts to suppress your stress response. Your stress hormone levels return to normal, but the battle to achieve homeostasis saps your energy. If the stress persists, your body may "fight back," staying in a constant state of arousal.

- *A stage of exhaustion:* In this phase, your ability to fight stress is gone. You're burned out, and your stress levels are constantly high. A chronic bath of stress chemicals damages your body—in particular, your cardiovascular system and your brain—and you experience memory problems, fatigue, or even clinical depression.

Before he came to me, Mason was in the "alarm reaction" stage and heading into resistance. While he still managed to cope most of the time, it took enormous energy. And things were getting worse for him—because, as Selye (1995) wrote, "No living organism can be maintained continuously in a state of alarm." Eventually, constant stress takes a greater toll—both physically and mentally. And that's what happened to the next two patients I'll talk about.

Mary and Anna: when alarm devolves into resistance or exhaustion

Mary, a 30-year-old schoolteacher, was in a downhill spiral when she first came to my office. The chronic anxiety she experienced when she needed to supervise a crowd of screaming kids on the playground or fight the rush-hour traffic on her way to work had pushed her into a state of resistance, and she was teetering on the edge of exhaustion.

When I first met Mary, she told me that she was chronically stressed and couldn't turn off the thoughts that raced through her mind. "I can never get out of my own head," she told me. She also suffered from colitis, had balance problems, and was often fatigued. Mary was aware that she would veer when walking because she attended to her right side of her body and suppressed her left side.

My evaluation of Mary showed that she was myopic, with a corrected acuity of 20/25 in each eye. The results of my testing indicated that Mary could fuse her two fields of view but relied mostly on tunnel vision. Her performance also indicated that her fixation was unstable. (This was actually an adaptive response, because she was able to view depth by making her left field of vision closer to an object than her right field of vision.) In addition, she exhibited a lack of resilience during the vergence testing, forcing herself to pay attention and eventually becoming fatigued.

Mary's problems are typical for controlling individuals who prefer fight to flight. In addition, people like Mary have figure–ground issues, focusing on figures rather than the background. (Put another way, they have difficulty "seeing the forest for the trees.")

Figure–ground problems often result in orientation and balance problems. In addition, they can cause a distorted awareness of self. Because Mary couldn't perceive the entire visual canvas of her world correctly, she had difficulty understanding her place in it.

In planning a patient's therapy, I choose "bottom-up" or "top-down" therapy depending on which approach allows a patient to reach a goal of relaxed attention faster. I decided to use a top-down approach in treating Mary—that is, to begin her therapy by addressing her conscious thoughts rather than challenging her unconscious feelings. I felt that if she tried disruptive lenses, she would likely fight and possibly go deeper into her tunnel. That, in turn, could lead to deeper psychological problems. So instead, I reduced the power of her prescription and gave her low-magnitude yoked prisms.

As I've noted, anxiety is global—and so is recovery from anxiety. Mary told me, "I believed that my anxiety might be related to vision but did not see the connection to the gastrointestinal issues. I was pleasantly surprised to see that once the therapy started working, my anxiety and GI symptoms both got better."

She added, "On my first visit, I noticed a change in my posture as well as the tightness in my chest. I also noticed my ability to sustain eye contact for a longer period of time." And when she wore her prism lenses, Mary told me, "I did not experience headaches as frequently, and my anxiety attacks were not as frequent. I also become more comfortable driving."

In my practice, this relaxed attention or "letting go" is the first goal in treatment. It's also the most crucial goal, because it sets the stage for real progress.

. . . .

The dancing patient

One of my favorite examples of "letting go" involved Matilda, a 49-year-old schoolteacher suffering from depression and anxiety. Within a few seconds after I gave her a pair of disruptive ambient lenses, she looked around the room, stood up, and started to dance. She yelled, "This is it! This is how I want to feel!"

Matilda still required months of therapy to fully overcome her visual problems. But in just the first few minutes, she was able feel a huge difference within her body—and that difference affected her emotions as well.

. . . .

At the time Mary came to my office, she was still able to battle her visual perceptual problems, which meant that she could function...barely. But in time, she would have fallen into Selye's final stage: exhaustion. This occurs when people collapse their tunnel vision into a "capsule" of space, and it's the stage Anna had devolved into when I first met her.

Anna, a 27-year-old woman, was working on a doctorate in electrical engineering. She'd always been a good student, but now her memory, cognition, and energy were taking a nosedive. As she studied for her final exams, she found herself re-reading the same paragraph several times and still not understanding what she'd read. She was unable to maintain a full work week and to handle simple tasks like managing emails and scanning papers.

My first insight into Anna's condition came when I learned that she was myopic and wore contacts that were changed every year. This is a common pattern for people whose careers require excessive close work.

In myopia, distant objects appear blurred because their images focus in front of the retina rather than on it. To correct this problem, we prescribe minus lenses that make the images of objects clearer. The catch is that these lenses also make images appear closer and smaller, perpetuating a person's myopic vision.

This is an important topic, so let me discuss it in more detail. At near point—that is, reading distance—the myopic reader has to move the book or paper closer, and this increases stress on the visual system. That's because moving the reading material closer forces the eyes to rotate further inward to maintain binocular vision (vergence). Because the vergence system is compromised in myopia, the reader compensates by tunneling (narrowing the field of vision), increasing stress and resulting in further myopia. It's a vicious cycle, and Anna was trapped in it.

Anna's history of vision problems began when she had surgery to correct strabismus at one year of age. The surgery made her look better, because her eyes no longer pointed in the wrong direction, but she still had issues in school throughout her life. She recalled writing letters backward, having poor listening skills, and finding sports and physical play unpleasant and stressful. However, she was extremely bright and was enough of a fighter to achieve high grades in college and get into a doctoral program.

But people with visual perception problems like Anna's can only fight for so long before their mounting anxiety forces them to give up. Eventually, Anna stopped reading, studying for school, and even watching television. She discontinued her medication for ADHD, and her day consisted of "cleaning and daydreaming." Given her history, it is no surprise that she was exhausted. Basically, she gave up.

When I examined Anna, I discovered that her prescription was much too strong to correct her myopia. Anna's lens correction had reduced the diameter of her visible field, contributing to her tunnel vision.

As Anna's educational demands had increased, so had the stress of dealing with her visual problems. She continued to react by compressing her visual field further and further. Eventually, her perceptual field was so constricted that she couldn't get enough information from what she read to comprehend it.

When I had Anna wear ambient yoked prisms, her posture improved dramatically. The base-up prisms also improved her breathing and reduced her tooth-grinding and sensory integration issues. However, she still had suppression problems.

My first inclination was to break Anna's suppression of one eye by giving her large-magnitude yoked prisms—the "hammer" approach I've talked about. However, she was too deep into her tunnel and wouldn't, or couldn't, respond to transformations in form, depth, and movement in her visual space. Luckily, I had one more trick up my sleeve: changing color.

I've often used complementary colors, such as yellow- and blue-tinted lenses, to bring out depth and improve reading for patients with learning problems. And it worked in this case as well. Anna sat and started to read for the first time in months.

Anna's school advisor, who accompanied her, asked why the lenses made such a big difference. I explained that colors are simply made up of different wavelengths, and these wavelengths move at different speeds. When you use complementary colors, you don't see them separately; rather, your perceptual system summates them into white and forms depth.

Anna's advisor said, "That's 'high definition'! How did you think of that?" He explained that high definition (HD) televisions rely on fusional overlap in which two wavelengths are projected to make images appear sharper.

Anna was scheduled to take her board exams three months later in November, and her advisor asked if she'd be ready for them. I replied, "No." He then asked, "How about in March?" I answered, "Ask me in December."

By December, Anna showed evidence of binocular vision, her vergence skills had improved markedly, and her acuity was 20/25. I was confident that she could pass her board exams after only four months of therapy. Better yet, she looked and felt like a new woman, her severe anxiety replaced by confidence and energy.

. . . .

Saving anxious, clumsy Jeff

Like Anna, many of my patients become anxious when they play sports because they're clumsy. Clumsiness is common in people with impaired ambient vision because balance and coordination are dependent on orientation—and good orientation requires vestibular and visual input, both of which are directly connected to the ambient visual pathway.

Jeff, a 45-year-old disc jockey, was a good example of how visual deficits can lead to clumsiness. But Jeff's clumsiness went beyond athletics, affecting both his career and his relationships.

Jeff's boss told him that he'd lose his job if he continued to knock over the equipment. Jeff was also anxious and depressed, a direct result of the stress caused by his visual problems, and his mental problems were severely affecting his job performance.

We designed a program for Jeff that helped him reorganize his attention to himself and to his world. As a result, his anxiety and depression eased and he became much less clumsy. Four months into therapy, he called me and said he wanted to thank me for saving his job and his marriage.

I understood how his therapy had helped with his job, but I told him I couldn't see the connection to his marriage. Laughing, he explained that when he walked with his wife in Manhattan, he often used to veer to his left and accidentally bump her into the street. At one point, she'd said, "One more time, and I will leave you." They now walk together in peace.

· ·

Seeing anxiety as a solution, not a problem

All of the patients I've discussed in this chapter had two things in common. First, they'd been diagnosed with the "mental disorder" of anxiety. And second, doctors had advised them to take anti-anxiety medications.

But for these people, anxiety wasn't a problem—it was a solution. Granted, it wasn't a very effective solution. But it was the best solution their brains could come up with.

Why did their brains make them feel anxious? Because their world truly *was* dangerous. A person with visual perceptual deficits is at far greater risk in a car or on a crowded sidewalk than a person with good vision. And when visual deficits lead a student like Anna to the verge of collapse, the brain's advice to go into full retreat makes perfect sense.

This is why addressing these people's anxiety with medications won't solve the problem. Instead, we need to step back and say: What problem is this person's brain attempting to solve by producing anxiety? If we discover that the answer lies in visual perceptual disturbances, we can plan an effective intervention. And in a short time, we can relieve these people of the burden of anxiety, empowering them to get back to school, back to work...or even back on the Tappan Zee.

VISUAL PERCEPTUAL IMPAIRMENT AND REDUCED EMPATHY

Is empathy an innate, unchangeable trait? And do some people—for instance, those with autism—simply lack the ability to feel empathy?

Here is another area in which I part ways with the mainstream scientific community. Many professionals believe that people with autism spectrum disorders or other emotional or affective disorders innately lack or have a diminished capacity for empathy. But in my practice, I've discovered that when I address these people's visual deficits, their ability to understand and respond to others' emotions often improves exponentially. Here are two examples, one involving a child and another involving an adult.

Justin: the boy who became a hugger

Justin came to my office with a diagnosis of autism spectrum disorder. He was six years old and displayed quite a few of the symptoms that define autism. As I "read" his behavior, I could see that many of these symptoms stemmed from delays in visual development.

For instance, Justin was unable to balance on one foot—a symptom of a visual spatial orientation delay. And when he walked, he needed to put his hand on the wall to guide him—a symptom of a visual spatial organization delay.

Justin's mother told me that he displayed fear and anxiety in large department stores, a setting that can be very confusing for people with visual deficits. And he didn't make eye contact, indicating a problem in centering his visual attention.

Using the Kaplan Nonverbal Battery (see Appendix II), I spotted more clues. When I asked Justin to stand on a rocking board and watch TV, he initially displayed fear and anxiety. But when I put base-up ambient yoked prisms on him, he relaxed and could easily attend to the TV. And when I asked Justin to wear the prisms as he walked to a mirror and looked at himself in it, his posture straightened. He could also attend to his image in the mirror while standing.

Next, I asked Justin to catch a ball without the lenses. His fear was obvious as he jerked his head back and failed to touch the ball until it hit his body. With the yoked prisms in place, however, he stood his ground and reached out and caught the ball. And afterward, he came over to me and hugged me tight—his actions speaking louder than his words.

Justin's mother wrote the following narrative to share the changes she saw as a result of Justin's visual management program. Notice that along with improvements in his language, cognitive skills, and self-help skills, he developed the ability to show empathy through both actions and words.

At the age of six years, our son, Justin, seldom spoke a clearly understandable word and full sentences were infrequent and not always related to a specific or appropriate circumstance. We did know, however, that he was a visual learner since he would often repeat a phrase or sentence from a video in a very appropriate situation.

It was our observation of our son that led us to believe he might have a visual disorder. He viewed books from the outer corner of his eye. He turned his head to the side while running and riding a tricycle or bicycle. He threw toys past the side of his head in order, perhaps, to watch them out of the corner of one eye.

In July of that year, we visited Dr. Melvin Kaplan for an evaluation. Justin was not particularly happy to be in the room and to be asked to perform tasks such as hitting a ball on a string, putting simple puzzles together, and walking on a balance beam. In fact, he left the room and ran upstairs crying three or four times during the evaluation. When asked to put donut circles on a pyramid without glasses, he threw the pieces around the room. With glasses, he immediately put the donuts on the pyramid. When asked to put wooden shapes in a puzzle board, he again performed the task without any problem.

Justin's first pair of glasses arrived two weeks after his evaluation. I gave them to him during lunch that day. He put them on and said, "I can see." Justin was still very limited verbally and seldom made such spontaneous statements.

Prior to that day, Justin had completed 12-piece puzzles on a backing, with the shape of the puzzle pieces carved into the backing, by matching puzzle pieces to their shapes on the backing. On that day, with glasses, he sat down and put together five puzzles quickly in succession. He placed the pieces around the edges, matching to colors and pictures for the first time. The next day he began putting two pieces together in his hands and completed the puzzles on the floor without any backing as a guide.

He stopped viewing books from the corner of his eye.

He began to run and ride a tricycle looking straight ahead.

Over the next couple of weeks, he stopped throwing toys past his head.

After about three weeks, he stopped wearing the glasses and did not want them. The changes in his behavior, however, remained.

In November, Justin returned to Dr. Kaplan for a re-evaluation. His reaction to trying the four types of lenses again indicated a difference in his behavior. When he got his second pair of glasses we were instructed to have him do some exercises to improve his awareness of himself and help him become bilateral.

The exercises were hitting a ball on a string with a rolling pin, walking on a tilted balance beam while holding a broomstick for balance, and rolling across the floor aiming parts of his body to roll over a beanbag.

Justin soon was hitting the ball 100 times with the rolling pin without missing. Walking on the balance beam was soon no challenge at all. Rolling on the floor to aim his body at a target did not interest him. However, he would often roll 25 to 30 times and seemed much calmer immediately following this exercise.

Within two days of receiving the second pair of glasses, Justin began taking his shirt off, touching people's faces, and hugging others more spontaneously. His eye contact also increased as he showed more interest in other people. He became less interested in his own solo play and more interested in watching what others were doing.

Over the five months since he began wearing his first pair of glasses, his speech has certainly increased noticeably in quantity. He now jabbers almost constantly and frequently throws out meaningful sentences.

In March, Justin would be seven years old. Needless to say, it was of considerable concern to us that Justin was as yet still soiling his pants for virtually all bowel movements. On December 31st of that same year, however, he used the toilet to move his bowels with total independence and great success...and has never again soiled his pants.

Today, March 23rd, Justin is spelling and writing words and numbers, reading sentences and books out loud, and answering social questions. He interacts wonderfully with his sisters and family.

Prior to January, he did not seem to have a decided preference for handedness. He is now using his left hand to write and eat, yet uses scissors successfully with his right hand.

His eye contact is that of a normal seven-year-old. His attention span allows up to two hours of continuous structure with only three- to five-minute breaks about every 30 minutes.

Justin, like many other people with autism, had symptoms that reflected a response to a confusing internal and external world. These included reduced empathy, hyperactivity, exaggerated feelings, and inappropriate responses to difficult tasks.

When I'm designing a visual management program for people like Justin, I address their issues by focusing on two questions: "What do you see?" and "What do you feel?" In cases where the person is nonverbal, I answer these questions by looking at how the person performs prior to treatment and what response I see when I apply yoked prisms.

In Justin's case, low-magnitude prisms allowed him to process information more efficiently. While he was probably unaware of the changes in his motor responses, the prisms gave him the ability to know where he was, allowing him to orient himself in space, reducing his level of anxiety, and giving him the ability to organize his world in reference to himself. And as a huge bonus, these changes helped him to relate more positively to the people around him.

The treatment protocol I developed for Justin has now been applied to additional patients of varying ages with autism spectrum disorders (research soon to be published). The results show a balancing of the autonomic nervous system and concomitant improvements in behavior and empathy, validating my clinical approach.

These results are not surprising. Human brain activity begins with visual perception, a sensible choice since so much of the brain's work is devoted to acquiring and integrating visual information. When we improve this visual perception, we dramatically change people's ability to respond to everything in their world—and that includes other people.

. . . .

ADHD and empathy

Attention is essential to empathy. Without an appropriate filtering mechanism, individuals become overwhelmed by the incredible amount of sensory information they receive and, based on my observations, they simply don't have enough energy left to perceive the needs and viewpoints of others.

So it makes sense that children diagnosed with attention deficit hyperactivity disorder (ADHD) often appear to lack empathy. This problem can become more pronounced as they age and school places increasing demands on them, further reducing their ability to process information in a short time and leaving them with less energy to focus on other people.

In children or adults with ADHD, impaired emotional empathy is just one symptom pointing to visual deficits. Others include poor short-term memory and an over-reliance on alternative sensory modalities (such as touch).

. . . .

Rick: the patient who became a better husband

A while ago, I received a call from a woman who'd attended a conference where I described how visual perceptual problems contribute to mental and emotional disorders. The woman explained that her husband was under treatment for depression, and she told me she was worried that their marriage would fall apart or he would lose his job.

Rick, the woman's husband, was in his late 40s. In addition to depression, his symptoms included anxiety and breathing issues. Fortunately, he agreed to make an appointment with me.

Rick's visual history started with his first pair of glasses at the age of 22, which was my initial clue that he had a visual perception disorder that was functional and not structural. (That's because the eye's structure finishes developing in the middle teens, not in adulthood. Thus, a structural problem would appear earlier.)

From a visual processing perspective, people with affective disorders often have issues with *spatial updating*. Spatial updating is the means by which we keep track of the location of objects in space. When it's working efficiently, our neural system maintains a consistent view as we shift our gaze, allowing us to maintain visual constancy. When it's not working efficiently, our vision is unstable.

Rick's deficits were clear from his performance on the Kaplan Star Test (see figure below).

Near Point Testing

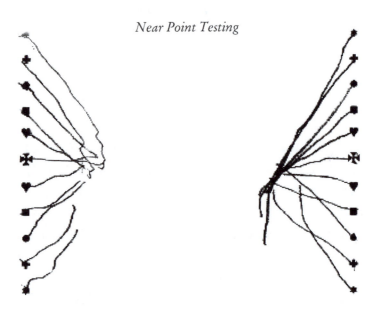

Rick's initial drawing

The results showed that Rick could not map his space world correctly. He was unable to maintain visual constancy, and his eyes could not lead his hands accurately. As a result, the model he drew at near point was extremely disorganized. (For more on the interpretations of this type of drawing, see Appendix I.)

At this point, my question was: Could Rick, in his late 40s, change his way of viewing the world, resulting in a higher level of perception and performance?

I approached the challenge using a top-down approach, applying large-magnitude disruptive prisms to make Rick consciously aware of the transformation of his visual world. Our recent study involving patients with autism spectrum disorders demonstrated that this light transformation affects the autonomic nervous system quickly.

The "awakening" induced by the light transformation allowed Rick to re-establish visual constancy and, as a result, to become much more efficient at spatial updating. His next drawing (below), which he completed nine months later, shows the remarkable change.

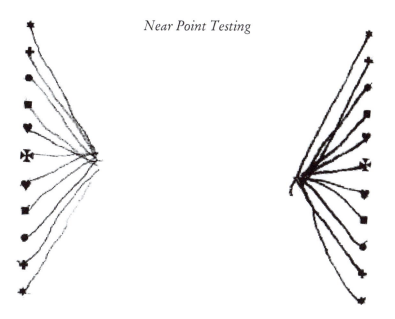

Near Point Testing

Rick's second drawing

Compared to the first drawing, Rick now exhibits spatial constancy and stability in both self-orientation and spatial organization.

Rick completed his program in 14 months. He no longer has yoked prisms in his prescription, and he reports that he feels much more "open" now. He's thriving at work and is back into photography, a passion of his. And his marriage—once on the rocks—is strong again.

At his final session, Rick asked Barbara, his therapist, a question: "Do you know what your program does?" She replied that it reprograms the way a person processes visual information. But Rick replied, "I believe that you teach empathy." Rick had noticed exactly what I've described in this chapter: that correcting visual deficits allows people to process information more quickly and efficiently—and this, in turn, frees up attention that they can focus on the interests and needs of the people around them.

10 VISUAL PERCEPTUAL IMPAIRMENT AND ISSUES WITH CONSCIOUSNESS AND MEMORY

To understand visual perception—as well as the often catastrophic effects of visual impairments—it's important to examine the role of consciousness.

People make the mistake of thinking that all aspects of perception are conscious. However, evidence suggests that perception becomes conscious at a late stage of information processing. When preconscious perception leads smoothly to conscious perception, we perform normally. When the mind needs to interfere due to a breakdown between preconscious and conscious perception, serious problems can occur, as the next patient's story shows.

. . . .

What is consciousness?

When you look at the pages in this book, you're conscious of them, directly experiencing images and words. In your private mental life, at the same time, you may be feeling some emotions and forming some thoughts. Together, these experiences make up "consciousness."

Psychologist Bruce Bridgeman (1992) wrote that consciousness is "the operation of the plan-executing mechanism, enabling behavior to be driven by plans rather than immediate environmental contingencies." As a clinician I would add these insights:

- The mind is not located in the head but instead embodied in the whole organism, which in turn is embedded in its environment. Thus, consciousness is a whole-body phenomenon.

- Cognition is a self-organizing process that spans and interconnects mind, body, and world.

- Humans are social creatures, and our cognitive emergence and consciousness are determined both by ourselves and by others.

Joanne: blowing the LSAT

Most people with visual perceptual problems suppress or alter their view of their spatial surroundings, and as a result they cannot integrate visual information rapidly. Because of this, they are unable to move quickly and easily from preconscious processing to conscious knowledge.

Joanne, who was referred to me by a friend many years ago, illustrates this point. Joanne had just graduated from college with grades high enough to earn her the honor of *summa cum laude*. However, she did quite poorly on the LSAT (Law School Admission Test) exam she needed to take to get into law school, and she was not accepted by any of the law schools to which she applied.

Joanne's visual examination revealed a visual processing disorder that enabled me to accurately predict the following problems:

- Joanne would have spatial orientation problems such as posture tilts, and a midline battle between the two halves of her body. These symptoms are associated with fear and anxiety.

- Joanne would have spatial organization problems—for instance, issues with balance, driving, and eye contact—due to poor depth perception. The pattern of her Kaplan Star profile was similar to that of other patients of mine who had suffered from emotional issues and learning problems such as poor reading comprehension.

The fact that Joanne had graduated with honors despite her visual impairment was remarkable. I was curious as to how she accomplished this feat. She told me that she was driven, and that if someone else studied for one hour, she would study for five hours or more. It confirmed for me what my testing had already told me: that she would do poorly on timed tests, because in that setting she just didn't have time to transition from preconscious processing (already knowing the answer) to conscious knowledge (figuring out the answer).

(By the way, this is a common occurrence for students with visual problems, and their parents often ask me for letters requesting that they receive extended time to take tests. I typically reply that this might get them through school, but it won't enable them to cope with real-world demands. So instead, I offer a limited-time letter, knowing that they won't need the extra time once we address their visual deficits.)

I demonstrated to Joanne that with her current glasses she could read, but her comprehension was quite poor. When I placed ambient yoked prisms over her glasses, however, she was able to read with speed and comprehension.

I developed a top-down program for Joanne, using disruptive lenses to make her consciously aware of her perception. My goal was to allow her to stabilize images on her retina, reducing the time she needed to organize her space world. This, in turn, reduced her need to pay attention to "where" the print was when she read, and allowed her to maximize her attention to the meaning, moving her from preconscious perception to conscious knowledge. Then I reintroduced her to tasks involving orientation, resulting in improved posture and gait and lessening the amount of attention she had to pay to her position in space.

Joanne retook her LSAT exam and did remarkably well. She entered a highly-ranked law school and ended up acing the bar exam the first time.

By the way, one question I'm often asked is, "Are gains like this lasting?" The answer is, "Largely, yes." However, some patients need an occasional "booster shot" of therapy in order to maintain their ability to move from preconscious perception to conscious knowledge. Joanne, for instance, completed her initial therapy back in 1989 and never had a recurrence of her symptoms. While she wore the prisms most of the time at first, she eventually wore them just while reading or using the computer. But she sometimes needs minor adjustments to her prisms, and she occasionally finds it helpful to do some of the exercises she learned during her therapy.

The role of consciousness in memory

Our current consciousness interacts with our memory, allowing us to analyze what we are perceiving. As a result, perception is not just a passive recording of sensory stimuli but an active mental reconstruction of the world in which we live. This is a two-way street, in which our memories color our current perceptions at the same time our current perceptions are building new memories.

The dominant model of information processing is the Stage Theory, set forth by Richard Atkinson and Richard Shiffrin in 1968. In this model, sensory memory and the environment provide us with many sources of information (light, sounds, smells, etc.). However, our brain can only understand this information if we can quickly transform it into a form of energy that can be passed on for additional memory processing. Memories need to be created in a short period of time: half a second for vision, and three to four seconds for hearing. This is why patients whose visual deficits prevent them from forming short-term memories will switch to auditory processing, which lasts much longer, even though they perceive less knowledge this way.

Visual memory flows in stages from sensory attention to perception and conscious meaning. Interference at different stages of visual information processing will result in "learning differences" which are also reflected in posture, attention, and emotion—the behavioral solutions that most clinicians see as "disorders."

Sensory memory is the earliest stage of memory. As I just mentioned, during this stage sensory information from the environment is stored for a brief period of time. In normal processing, information next passes through the stage of short-term memory (action memory). Many of our short-term memories are quickly forgotten. But if we attend to this information, it progresses to become part of our long-term memory. A key role of a visual management program is to identify and correct the glitches in this process so that individuals can effectively process the information they need in order to learn, make decisions, and interact easily with other people.

Looking at consciousness from a different angle

When I see patients with visual deficits, I don't just evaluate their ability to move from unconscious perception to conscious thought in their daily lives. In addition, I assess their awareness that they actually *have a visual problem*. That's because unless they're consciously aware of how their visual impairments affect them, they won't be motivated to change.

Even when patients have significant visual impairments, they—and not I—decide if therapy is necessary. So my job is simply to show them the problems a visual impairment is causing them, so they can determine how significant this impairment is in their lives.

To do this, I first profile patients and explain to them how I believe problems in information processing are impacting their lives academically, professionally, and socially. Next, I illustrate the problems they have with perception and performance—for instance, by having them perform a ball-catching task with and without prisms. And finally, I demonstrate solutions that will raise their level of adaptation.

Often, patients are immediately motivated to start therapy. However, some patients are so accustomed to their own solutions that it's hard for them to see the need to change. Here are the stories of two patients who were in this position.

Sarah and Percy: two patients, two different decisions

Seventeen-year-old Sarah's younger brother was just finishing a visual management program at my office, and his parents were thrilled with his progress. One day, Sarah's father asked if he could speak with me about his daughter as well.

Sarah was at the top of her class, but she lacked friends and social graces. She never complained about any vision issues, but her dad was worried about her isolation and wondered if my program would spark a change in her social behavior.

I examined Sarah, and the results indicated that she operated spatially in a tightly restricted tunnel. Her view of the world was two-dimensional, and her unstable saccadic eye movements were causing poor eye contact, a lack of depth perception, and balance issues.

The first stage in my protocol was to stimulate a conscious awareness of the perceptual delays that were compromising Sarah's social interactions. I asked her to stand on one foot, catch a ball, read a paragraph, and so on, first without and then with prisms.

As Sarah completed each task, her father and I were excited by her postural changes in response to the prisms. But when I asked Sarah to tell me what differences she felt when she did the tasks without and then with the prisms, her answer was always the same: "I don't know." Her level of awareness was so low that she couldn't move from preconscious to conscious memory of her actions.

To me, this suggested that she was unlikely to benefit from therapy. In private, I told her father that Sarah wasn't a candidate for my program at that time. She needed to hit bottom before she'd be motivated to want to change. He said, "I saw all those positive changes." I said, "We both did. But Sarah didn't."

I told Sarah's father to go home and talk with her about what had occurred during her evaluation. This, I explained, would help her become aware of the changes we had seen.

Sarah's father was encouraged, and the next day I received a call from him, telling me that Sarah was ready to participate in a visual management program. He shared with me how this turnaround came about. He told me he'd said to Sarah, "How come you couldn't explain what happened in Dr. Kaplan's office?" Her answer was, "I couldn't answer him with language, but I can write it out for you." She wrote verbatim exactly what occurred from the time she entered my office until she left. And she followed her description with these words: "I would like to try the program because I am tired of being so alone."

As Sarah went through her program, the change in her social behavior was swift and remarkable. On her fifth visit, we were delighted when she entered with a smile and a greeting to everyone in the office.

While some patients, like Sarah, become aware that their problems are debilitating, others decide that their current adaptations—even if not optimal—are acceptable. In general, these patients have a high level of resilience and are experiencing problems that do not cause them extreme difficulty socially, academically, or in their careers.

Percy was one of these patients. Until his college days, Percy always had good visual acuity. However, in his freshman year, he began to see double when reading. He adapted by using one eye for near-point acuity and the other for seeing in the distance. This worked until he reached 52 years of age and started to have problems seeing clearly for reading. He visited his ophthalmologist, who told him he had age-related presbyopia and needed magnification for reading. The doctor gave him a prescription for bifocals.

From the very first day, Percy complained about the difficulty of using his new glasses. Percy's wife had heard about me, and she told him to make an appointment with me.

After finishing my consultation, I explained to Percy that he had a functional visual issue that he solved by alternating his eyes when he viewed things at different distances. The bifocals, although helping him to see clearly, were creating double vision when he read. So he had two options:

1. He could enter a visual management program that would entail two years of therapy.

2. He could return to using one eye for far viewing and the other for near viewing, with one eyeglass lens designed to help him read easily.

Percy chose option 2, which satisfied his needs. He felt comfortable with his new glasses, which allowed him to see with depth perception and to read faster with improved comprehension.

In each of these cases—Sarah's and Percy's—I encouraged my patients to make their own decisions. And both made wise choices, based on their conscious perception of their visual issues, the solutions they had developed for dealing with them, and the impact that vision therapy could have on their lives.

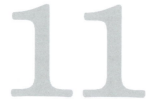

11 VISUAL PERCEPTUAL IMPAIRMENT AND MOTION SICKNESS

For people who experience motion sickness, traveling by car, plane, train, or boat can be an utterly miserable experience. But yoked prism lenses can often dramatically reduce or even eliminate nausea and other symptoms of motion sickness.

In 1975 I published a paper titled "An optometric approach to motion sickness" (Kaplan 1975), based on reports I heard from parents of children who'd previously displayed symptoms of motion sickness, including nausea, dizziness, and in extreme cases tinnitus (ringing in the ears). When I placed base-up ambient yoked prisms on these children, their symptoms disappeared.

In reviewing these cases, I detected a pattern of optometric measurements that seemed to profile individuals with a predisposition for motion sickness. And clinically, I noticed that children with motion sickness often had an "exotropic" alignment of the eye (in which one or both eyes turn outward). They compensated by alternating their fixation from field to field, and they typically displayed reading problems and other academic issues.

In time, I came to realize that these abnormal reflexive eye movements, an adaptive strategy used to make images stabilize on the retina, were the cause of these children's motion sickness. As I mentioned earlier, the vestibulo-ocular reflex (VOR) is a reflex eye movement that stabilizes images on the retina during head movements by producing eye movements in the direction opposite to the head movements, thus preserving the image of the visual field. In these children, abnormal eye movements likely caused the VOR to send false information about where their bodies were in space.

Research shows that motion sickness can stem from a rivalry between the visual and vestibular systems (Oman 1990). The visual aspect of the VOR is associated with the parasympathetic (peripheral) nervous system, while the vestibular aspect is associated with the sympathetic (central) nervous system. If the visual and vestibular systems compete rather than cooperate—which is what happens when the brain is getting false visual information—vertigo will result.

Studies show that visual information is more important than vestibular input in causing motion sickness. However, dizziness, fatigue, and nausea can arise as a result of problems in the vestibular system and/or the visual system. In the vestibular system, the symptoms are referred to as the *Coriolis effect*, and in vision they are known as the *pseudo-Coriolis effect*.

Fortunately, symptoms of motion sickness stemming from either visual or vestibular problems often resolve completely when I apply prism lenses combined with a program of vision therapy. Since writing my 1975 paper, I've successfully treated many children with motion sickness—and many adults as well. Here are four typical cases.

Tony: motion sickness in the car

Tony, an eight-year-old whose parents brought him to my office, had unstable eye movements that left him with learning difficulties, anxiety, and motion sickness. His parents learned over time to keep Tony's car trips short and to avoid placing him in the back seat of the car because this aggravated his symptoms.

Tony was responding very well to base-up yoked prisms along with therapy. His reading improved, he went from failing grades to As, and his nausea, headaches, and anxiety subsided.

Tony's parents were encouraged enough to take a car trip to Grandma's house some 30 miles away. Their van had a video screen and books and games to keep Tony and his siblings happy.

Tony's mother noticed how content Tony was, but she herself was starting to feel symptoms of motion sickness. So she asked Tony if she could try his glasses on for a short time. Fifteen minutes later, she was symptom-free, but Tony's motion sickness had come back with a vengeance and lasted until they reached Grandma's house.

Candice: motion sickness on the water

Candice, the mother of a child in therapy, mentioned to me that she wasn't looking forward to the Fourth of July holiday because her husband was an avid sailor and she suffered from motion sickness.

I asked her, "Would you like to try an experiment?" Because the holiday was only a few days away, I didn't have time to get the laboratory to add prisms to her existing prescription. However, I did have yoked prisms without refractive correction available for training sessions. I gave her a pair of plano 5-diopter base-up yoked prisms to wear when she was out at sea.

I explained that although she was quite near-sighted, she could do fine without her glasses as she and her husband sailed from New York to Martha's Vineyard. "Your most crucial need during your trip," I said, "is not to see objects clearly, but to be able to control the movement of the boat and of the environment. The prisms will allow you integrate what you see and how you feel."

Candice was skeptical, but she decided to give it a try. Later, when she brought her son in for a therapy session, she was smiling from ear to ear. Excitedly, she told me that the prism lenses had given her the best vacation she'd ever had. She'd experienced no signs of motion sickness at all.

She made an appointment, and I prescribed lenses for refraction in concert with yoked prisms. Many years after moving to Florida, she makes an annual trek to my office for follow-up appointments.

Bruce and Valerie: two cases of "disembarking vertigo"

A nephew of mine who lived on the island of Nantucket called me one evening. Bruce made his living on the water, lobstering and scalloping. He told me that he was being treated at Massachusetts General Hospital for symptoms of disequilibrium, including dizziness and light-headedness.

Doctors eventually diagnosed Bruce with a vestibular system disorder that has a very fancy name: *mal de débarquement* syndrome. People with this condition feel fine while they're on a plane or boat, but begin experiencing vertigo when they get off. Symptoms can last for months or years and sometimes are permanent.

Bruce's symptoms filled him with anxiety and interfered with his work and social activities. After three months of treatment, his symptoms and the depression that followed had not let up. Then he thought back to when we spent summers together at his parents' home in Humarock, and he remembered my conversations about using prisms and therapy to treat visual disorders. He asked if I could examine him in hopes of finding a solution.

Bruce's evaluation revealed the typical pattern of symptoms I'd identified in people with motion sickness. After examining him, I created a visual management program for him involving yoked prisms and a top-down (conscious-to-unconscious) therapy approach.

Six months later, Bruce was symptom-free at work. Socially, he became involved in local politics and could stand in front of an audience and speak confidently. At present he is captaining a yacht and is delighted with his change of fortune.

After this experience, I knew exactly how to proceed when a good friend called and told me that his wife, Valerie, who has high-functioning autism, was suffering from similar symptoms. The following narrative was written by Valerie following her treatment.

On New Year's Eve, just as the year was changing from 2012 to 2013, I was aboard a cruise ship with my family in the Caribbean to celebrate my mother's eightieth birthday. I had never been on a cruise before, and before embarking on the ship, I had trepidation about going on the weeklong journey. This is because of a sensory integration condition I have that is associated with my autism.

In the past, short trips on smaller boats, such as a sailing excursion with friends, left me with "sea legs." Though my symptoms of imbalance and rocking sensations would pass within a few days, I avoided boats as much as I could.

A long trip at sea with my family, for a full week, was daunting to consider. This is because I experience vestibular vulnerability, particularly when I am under emotional or physical stress. During such times, the ground below me unexpectedly "drops" beneath my feet, or I experience wavelike sensations that cause me to stumble or feel nauseated, as if I were on a boat. Such sensory dysregulation, experienced by many of us with autism, is often accompanied with or followed by deep fatigue that can be debilitating, limiting our activities and the ability to be in a variety of environments.

I wanted very much to be a part of the family celebration, so I went on the cruise. I had a wonderful time, too. I didn't feel seasickness and enjoyed every moment. But life changed dramatically after I disembarked. I began experiencing severe disequilibrium, as I never had before. Back at home, at night, my bed would rock so much that I couldn't tell whether it was my vestibular problem, or if we were having an earthquake. (I was living in Southern California at the time.) A few days went by, and I hoped the symptoms would pass. A week went by, then two, then three weeks. I was exhausted. I wasn't able to work full days at my office, and on some days I couldn't work at all. When I did try to do tasks on the computer, my system would become triggered, and I'd find myself home in bed for one to two days waiting for my fatigue to dissipate enough for me to go back to work.

In February, I went to a top ear/nose/throat consultant in San Diego, who was also a neurologist and specialized in inner ear and balance conditions. Tests run at the hospital showed no indication of brain tumors or hearing loss, and I also tested out of vertigo, which is a condition very different from the one I have.

I was provided with various diagnoses, from disequilibrium, to inner ear damage due to a viral infection, to what's called *mal de débarquement* syndrome. I was also told that it was unclear whether my condition would ever improve, and that if it did, the symptoms would never go away entirely. This was hard news.

I was placed on a rigorous regimen of therapies that were physically based, such as daily use of a rowing machine while staring, from different angles, at a point in front of me. I also attended physical therapy and began taking private yoga classes three days each week. These yoga sessions provided me with temporary relief, so that I could do some work. Meanwhile, very little changed. On hard days, walking down the street, I looked as if I were drunk. I easily stumbled or fell off curbs while crossing the street. Inside buildings, I had to be seated facing a window and looking out, and I could not make eye contact with the people I was speaking to, because my symptoms would become impossible. Instead, if I fixed my gaze outside, I could manage a conversation with difficulty. Rooms with no windows, stairwells, and other enclosed environments were the very worst places I could be. I avoided these entirely.

By late March 2013, in spite of all my therapies, I was not seeing progress. The ear/nose/throat consultant suggested that I would eventually habituate to my symptoms and learn to live with them. This was distressing to me. I had to face the possibility that I would never be able to work at the capacity I was used to and that I would not be able to be in many environments. These realities began to affect my emotional well-being. I was becoming depressed and spent a great deal of time in bed. The days become long and grey. When I could work half of a day, I had to rest the remainder of the day and through the evening until bedtime. I have never been so bedridden in my life, and never so scared. I saw friends less and less. I spent a lot of time alone.

I work in the autism field. I travel a lot for my work and during this period, I had to cancel all my trips. I knew that something had to change. My livelihood and happiness were at risk, and although I was putting accommodations into place at work and at home, I didn't feel I had exhausted the possibilities for finding improvement.

That's when I decided to finally brace myself and get onto an airplane. I went to see Dr. Mel Kaplan at the Center for Visual Management in Tarrytown, New York. Dr. Kaplan had been successfully treating children with autism who experienced vestibular and proprioceptive problems like mine by prescribing prism lenses for them to wear. The visual and vestibular sense systems are profoundly connected. That's why, for example, whenever I worked on the computer, my visual processing would in turn affect my sense of balance. The first thing Dr. Kaplan told me when I arrived at his office was that my neurologist in San Diego was treating my condition as a "hardware problem" and that he was going to treat it differently, as a "software problem."

The prism lenses he prescribed arrived in the mail a couple of weeks later. I began wearing them, and I also began doing the exercises that Dr. Kaplan's office sent to me via email. I was tracking my progress. In fact I had begun collecting data on myself months before I went to be evaluated at Dr. Kaplan's office, taking daily measurements of my level of fatigue, level of rocking sensation and imbalance, as well as how much I slept each day. I also began taking data on the exercises I was given.

Although the data never amounted to a study because of its obvious subjectivity, the shift in my ability to sustain work for longer periods of time was real, as was my ability to be in environments I was previously avoiding because my symptoms would worsen. Within the first week, I found I had more energy in general. By the second week, my sense of imbalance and the "drunken walk" and bumping into tables and corners began to subside. The improvement was gradual yet obvious. Most of all, the awful fatigue that kept me in bed began to dissipate.

Because of the lenses, I was able to organize and attend important briefings and make a presentation, under very stressful circumstances, at the United Nations in early April on World Autism Awareness Day. I did not fail to mention Dr. Kaplan's important work while I was there. In addition to the prism lenses and exercises, I continued to do my other therapies as well. They contributed to my physical fitness and I felt they were supportive to the treatment I was undergoing.

Another dramatic change I must report on was *what* I saw and *how* I saw with the prism lenses. Basically, they opened a door to me that I had not known was closed. I had always assumed that I saw what people call "three-dimensionality." However, with the lenses, the world suddenly had more depth than I had ever known. Dr. Kaplan explained that the stress of processing information without this dimensionality affects the vestibular systems of people with autism. It's why children can't learn, why adults have difficulty becoming employed or maintaining employment. Not only was this revelatory for me, the world itself had become so much more beautiful and rich to behold. I saw trees on a horizon, with more trees at a further distance and could, for the first time, discern the distance between the layers in my visual field. I went through my day "oohing and ahhing," as I like to say, at the beauty around me.

It has now been eight months since I first saw Dr. Kaplan for my evaluation and twelve months since I disembarked from the cruise that rocked my world (pun intended). By August of 2013, four months after I visited Dr. Kaplan, my daily symptoms were gone. Only on occasional days now do I feel a shadow of the past, and it's usually when I'm very tired or feeling some emotional stress. I continue to wear my lenses and to do the eye exercises. With time, I will no longer need the lenses at all. For me, the most important message I wish to share in this account is that adults with autism like myself may find great benefit from prism lenses in the way I have. In my own work in the autism community, I am committed to informing others about this most useful and promising intervention that saved my livelihood and my happiness. (Valerie Paradiz, Ph.D, Director, Autistic Global Initiative, Autism Research Institute)

Doctors tend to view motion sickness and *mal de débarquement* as separate clinical entities. However, the symptoms of motion sickness are the same as the symptoms of *mal de débarquement*, and clinically should be treated in the same way.

Typically, the medical community addresses these symptoms with medication, physical therapy, psychotherapy, or surgery. However, these approaches frequently are ineffective. As a result, people with these problems suffer greatly or even—in many cases of *mal de débarquement*—become crippled for life.

My question for the medical community is: Why not treat these patients instead with a program of vision therapy that is non-invasive, has no medical side effects, and, above all, is clinically proven to work? There is nothing to lose, and—for patients whose symptoms are annoying, upsetting, or even catastrophic—there is everything to gain.

Section 4

CONCLUSION

12

A LOOK AT
THE RESEARCH

Past, Present, and Future

As the remarkable case studies in this book prove, vision therapy using prism lenses can have a profound effect on patients with learning disabilities, emotional disorders, cognitive problems, movement disorders, and behavioral problems. Yet research on this powerful approach is still in its infancy. It is my hope that this book will inspire researchers to explore the promise of this intervention in greater depth.

For my part, I have been involved in a number of studies conducted over three decades. These studies confirm that there is a high prevalence of visual problems in people with emotional, behavioral, cognitive, movement, and learning disorders. In addition, they strongly support the efficacy of using prism lenses in combination with a visual management program to treat these individuals. In this chapter, I look at my own findings and discuss new avenues for professionals to pursue in the future.

My initial research with Dr. Flach

In 1975 a 23-year-old woman, Rickie Flach, came to my office. Rickie had been in and out of institutions for many years. Her father, Frederic Flach M.D., a psychiatrist, had heard about my holistic approach to vision and felt it was worth a try.

Rickie was my first patient with a diagnosis of schizophrenia. The results of my exam were quite compelling. Her initial acuity without lenses was 20/30, well within normal range. A retinoscopic exam indicated a low hyperopia (far-sightedness) with normal color vision.

When I asked Rickie to sit and visually track a wand as I moved it in different directions, her eye movements were slightly saccadic—probably no different from what I would see in a typical patient with learning differences. But when I asked her to stand and repeat the activity, her eyes jumped all over the place. I didn't expect this to happen, and I stopped and put up the Snellen chart to retest her visual acuity. This time, it was 20/200. In effect, she was considered clinically blind.

I sat Rickie down and placed base-up yoked prisms on her, and she immediately calmed down. When I retested her, her acuity had returned to 20/30.

Next, I asked Rickie to complete the Van Orden Star (a pencil-and-paper test of visual function, which I later modifed as the Kaplan Star Test; see Appendix I). She drew a disorganized star of unequal vergence and below the line.

I sat Dr. Flach down and explained that my findings indicated that Rickie had serious problems with spatial orientation (indicated by her anxiety when standing and tracking) and spatial organization (indicated by her mapping pattern on the Van Orden Star). He looked at me and asked, "Can you help her?" My answer was, "Visually or emotionally?" He replied, "Any way you can."

I designed a treatment program for Rickie. During that time she also underwent nutritional therapy and counseling at another facility, where a dedicated staff ensured that she did her vision therapy exercises.

The results were remarkable. Rickie, who was terrified and almost nonfunctional when she first came to my office, became a happy, successful woman. She married, had children, and had a successful career as a nurse.

Fred and Rickie wrote a book, titled *Rickie* (Flach 1990), which describes the astonishing changes in her life as a result of her visual management program. Dr. John Ratey's book *A User's Guide to the Brain* (2002) also describes the transformative effects of Rickie's therapy.

Meeting Rickie and Dr. Flach was a turning point in my career. Fred and I started a long professional relationship, and I was able to help many of his patients. In addition, we conducted two research studies.

In 1983, Dr. Flach and I published a paper, "Visual perceptual dysfunction in psychiatric patients," in the *Journal of Comprehensive Psychiatry* (Flach and Kaplan 1983). In this study we examined 57 patients, 48 of them with diagnosed psychiatric disorders. We found that 32 of these patients had significant visual perceptual problems, primarily affecting spatial organization and/or orientation. Patients with major depressive disorders, schizophrenia, or alcoholism were the most likely to have visual perceptual problems. We also discovered that visual perceptual problems were more common in patients who'd been ill for more than six months, and in those who were socially withdrawn or had experienced difficulties achieving in school or keeping a job.

Several years after completing this study, Dr. Flach and I, along with several other colleagues, completed a second study titled "Visual perceptual dysfunction: schizophrenic and affective disorders vs. controls." This study appeared in the *Journal of Neuropsychiatry and Clinical Neurosciences* (Flach *et al.* 1992).

In our second study we used standardized tests, supplemented by the Visual Skills Test and Kaplan Star Test, to evaluate visual perception in 26 hospitalized patients with schizophrenia, 23 hospitalized patients with affective disorder, and 60 control subjects. We found that the mentally ill patients differed significantly from the control group. For example, both groups of patients exhibited significant anomalies in both pursuit tracking (in which the eyes follow a target) and vergence tracking (in which the eyes should smoothly and simultaneously turn inward to view close-up objects).

Research into autism

In more recent years I began focusing much of my attention on autism, after my creation of the Kaplan Nonverbal Battery (see Appendix II) made testing of nonverbal patients possible. Between 1996 and 2012 my colleagues and I published a range of studies exploring the incidence of visual problems in autism and the effects of prism lenses.

In the first study in 1996, titled "Postural orientation modifications in autism in response to ambient lenses" and published in *Child Psychiatry and Human Development* (Kaplan, Carmody and Gaydos 1996), we evaluated the response of 14 children with autism to yoked prism lenses. We found that the lenses immediately improved posture, head tilt, and ball-catching abilities.

In a 1998 study titled "Behavioral changes in autistic individuals as a result of wearing ambient transitional prism lenses," published in *Child Psychiatry and Human Development* (Kaplan, Edelson and Seip 1998), my colleagues and I evaluated 18 subjects who wore either prism lenses or plain glasses for several months. As we predicted, we observed a significant decrease in behavioral problems after participants wore the prism lenses for two months. This finding was consistent with the phenomenon called "visual capture," in which ambient prism lenses lead to consolidation of the visual system. Because participants did not receive vision therapy to make this consolidation permanent, their behavioral improvement was not lasting.

In a later paper, titled "Strabismus in autism spectrum disorder" and published in 1999 in *Focus on Autism and Other Developmental Disabilities* (Kaplan, Rimland and Edelson 1999), we reported evidence that vision problems are epidemic in autism. Our survey of 7640 families found that 20 percent of autistic children had been identified with strabismus. And a more sensitive clinical examination of 34 individuals with autism found a 50 percent rate of strabismus (failure of the eyes to align correctly, making it impossible for a person to form an accurate composite image). In comparison, only two percent to four percent of the general population has strabismus.

Finally, in a 2012 study titled "Effects of ambient prism lenses on autonomic reactivity to emotional stimuli in autism" and reported at the International Meeting for Autism Research (IMFAR) (Sokhadze *et al.* 2012), my colleagues and I studied 21 children with autism as they watched scenes from a movie while wearing yoked prisms or plain glasses. Measuring their heart rate, heart rate variability, and skin conductance levels, we detected lower heart rates and increased skin conductance responses in the prism group during viewing, indicating increased attention to audio-visual stimuli. In addition, we detected higher skin conductance in the group wearing prisms when they watched "emotionally loaded" scenes, indicating increased arousal and attentiveness to the emotional content of these scenes. Based on our findings, we concluded that improved ambient vision has a positive impact on autonomic function and behavior in children with autism, and has the potential to ameliorate autistic behaviors and improve communication.

Future directions

Taken together, our research findings and my own clinical experience make two points very clear. First, visual impairment is epidemic in individuals with cognitive, behavioral, learning, movement, or emotional problems. And second, vision therapy with yoked prisms is one of the most effective tools we have to help these people.

At this point, there are many intriguing questions for researchers and clinicians to investigate. For example:

- Can the Kaplan Star Test (see Appendix I) and Visual Skills Test be used to predict reading disorders?

- Can yoked prisms often replace patching or surgery in treating idiopathic toe-walking and/or idiopathic scoliosis?

- Can yoked prisms be an effective tool for treating affective disorders?

For the sake of the millions of people currently suffering from the effects of undiagnosed visual perceptual disorders, I hope that a new generation of researchers will be eager to pursue these questions. And I hope, too, that a new generation of clinicians will be open to exploring the benefits of vision therapy for their patients. As the stories in this book show, this simple and powerful intervention can dramatically change the life of a child or adult for the better—forever.

Afterword

One question I ask my patients after I describe my program of visual management is "Did I make myself clear?" And to help ensure that my message in this book is clear as well, here is a final look at the core principles of the Kaplan method of visual management:

- Symptoms are not the problem, but rather clues that can steer the clinician to a solution.

- Visual processing problems affect not just vision but also mood, emotion, cognition, behavior, and posture. To understand visual perceptual problems, clinicians must look not just at the eyes but at the whole person and how that person interacts with the world.

- A label is not a diagnosis. Many people labeled as depressed, anxious, emotionally troubled or learning-disabled are actually suffering from visual perceptual problems. Visual problems can also play a large role in severe disorders such as schizophrenia and autism.

- Visual perceptual problems stem from missed developmental steps. The more steps an individual has missed, the more likely the person is to have severe visual perceptual problems and resulting behavioral and emotional problems.

- Visual perceptual problems involve orientation (difficulty in perceiving the position of the body in space) and organization (difficulty in correctly perceiving the surrounding environment). Yoked prisms transform the light entering the eyes, encouraging the eyes to move together in a uniform manner. As a result, these prisms cause a remapping of a person's visual surroundings, improving spatial organization and orientation.

- Yoked prisms "capture" improved performance. Therapy permanently consolidates these improvements.

- The *perceptual* model of vision can be summed up as: *space × time = knowledge*. In this model, *space* relates to the external world and *time* involves the internal processing we need to perform in order to gain information from this world and process it in our mind. The more quickly we can do this, the more knowledge we can acquire. And the more knowledge we can acquire, the more successfully we can navigate our world. The goal of visual management is to allow individuals to process more information about their space in less time, reducing stress and improving performance.

THE KAPLAN STAR TEST AND THE KAPLAN NONVERBAL BATTERY

The Kaplan Star Test

Throughout these chapters, I have extolled the predictive power of the Kaplan Star Test. This test is a mapping of the mind's orientation and organization of information processing. By viewing the test results, I can identify my patients' problems with an extremely high degree of accuracy.

Using the Kaplan Star

The instrument of choice for this test is the Correct-Eye-Scope with the transilluminated back. The Scope has an adjustable shaft with a Brewster stereoscope attached. The shaft marks dictate the visual distance to which the subject will attend.

The test itself consists of a white translucent paper with two columns of figures, such as a star and a cross. In the first segment of the test, columns are composed of 11 figures placed 140mm apart, for far-point testing. In the second segment of testing, the shaft is adjusted to the near-point setting. A new test sheet is given, with the same columns of figures now 95mm apart.

Figure 1 below shows what the Kaplan Star looks like. It is modified from the original Van Orden Star, allowing me to test both near- and far-point demands.

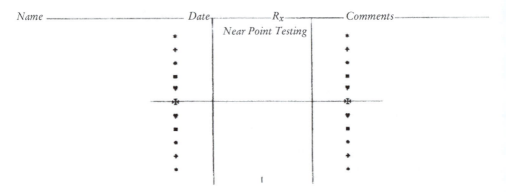

Name ———————————— Date ——— R$_x$ ——— Comments ———

Near Point Testing

Figure 1: The Kaplan modification of the Van Orden Star

To administer the test, direct the patient to sit in front of the instrument and look through the eyepiece. Ask the patient, "How many columns of figures do you see?" If the answer is "Two," ask, "Can you see both columns at the same time, or do they appear one at a time?" If the answer is the former, direct the patient to take two same-size pencils, one in each hand. Guide the patient to hold the pencils so as to write with both simultaneously. Ask the patient to place a pencil point on the center cross of each column—right pencil on the right cross, left on the left. Now ask, "Can you see both pencil points at the same time?" If yes, have the patient draw simultaneous lines, one toward the other, until the pencil points look as if they're touching. Next, place the left pencil on the top figure of the left column, and the right pencil on the bottom figure of the right. As before, the two pencils are to be brought toward each other until they appear to touch. The procedure is repeated with successive figures until the star pattern is complete.

Interpreting Kaplan Star patterns

Figure 2 below shows what a normal Kaplan Star pattern looks like. The "A" lines create an illusion of a frontal plane. The "B" line creates an illusion of the sagittal plane. The As are associated with postural alignment of the body. The Bs are associated with depth perception of the world.

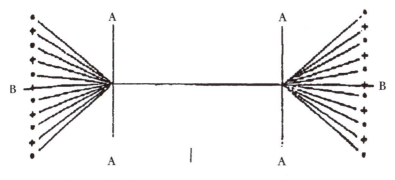

Figure 2: A normal Kaplan Star pattern

Execution of this pattern, while straightforward and simple, requires the individual to rapidly and accurately interpret what he or she sees, generate a motor response, and maintain attention throughout. The appearance of this star pattern is, fundamentally, a predictor of the patient's spatial behavior. It reveals the way the person responds to internal and external constraints and depicts his or her particular version of homeostasis.

If the patient's Star drawing shows apices above or below primary gaze or the target midline, as shown in Figure 3, this is evidence of errors in vergence.

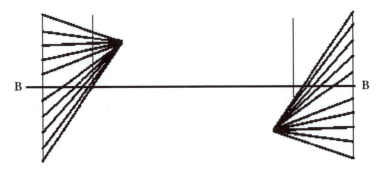

Figure 3

The next pattern, shown in Figure 4, denotes constraints of the peripheral–central relationship. My interpretation suggests that this pattern results when central demands supersede peripheral demands, and an individual selects a space location closer to himself or herself. The visible space world is rotated about the horizontal axis, bringing the sagittal plane closer, and directing the apices above the line. This type of individual will display behaviors associated with tunnel vision.

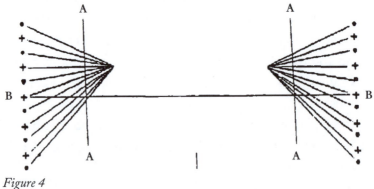

Figure 4

Figure 5 also represents constraints in the peripheral–central relationship. In this relationship, peripheral demands supersede focal (central) demands. The visible space world is again rotated about the horizontal axes, but here, the sagittal plane appears further away, and apices appear above the line. This pattern is usually associated with individuals who have increased near-point activity and visual stress.

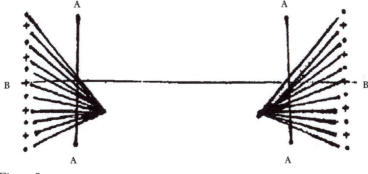

Figure 5

Figure 6a displays constraints in the peripheral–central relationship that are manifested by disorganization of the visual system. The apices are poorly formed. Either they do not form an apex, as seen on the left side, or they form a fan shape, as seen on the right. These patients usually present a peripheral bias with no perceptual constancy. There may be an emotional component to their visuo-spatial distortion.

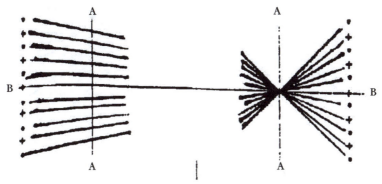

Figure 6a

In a study composed of 60 emotionally disturbed patients at the Westchester Medical Center and 60 control subjects, we compared far-point Van Orden Star patterns. There was a significant difference between the schizophrenic patients and the control subjects. Typically, the schizophrenic subjects showed a crossing, fan-like presentation on the right side, and no apex formation on the left (P=0.003). Compare the top pattern (patients) and bottom pattern (controls) in Figure 6b.

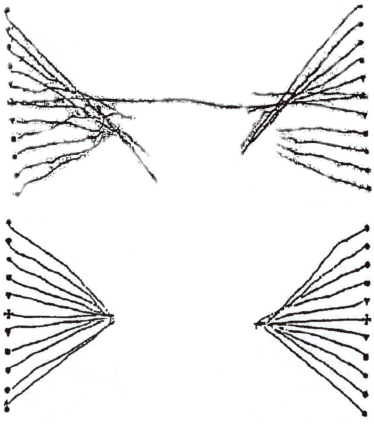

Figure 6b

Figure 7 shows constraints in the peripheral–central relationship, which show up as disorientation in the apices. These constraints are functional warps, and they can be seen in physical performance as well as in a pencil-and-paper manifestation. For instance, when the patient is walking, a foot may toe in rather than point straight ahead. The star pattern apices may be clearly formed, but they differ in linear length. The pattern is rotated about the vertical axis, a projection of a body image that is rotated around the mid-body axis. The subject's perception of his or her space world makes the frontal plane closer on the larger apex side than on the shorter apex side.

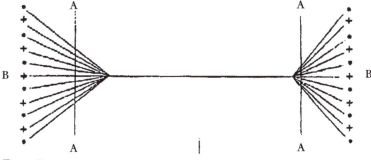

Figure 7

Figure 8 represents constraints in the peripheral–central relationship that imply disorientation and disorganization. The star has poorly formed apices. There is no apex on the left, and the right side forms a fan. There are many variations of this rendition, with apices being unequal along the frontal plan, or positioning above or below the midline. These star patterns are usually seen in individuals with concomitant visual and emotional issues.

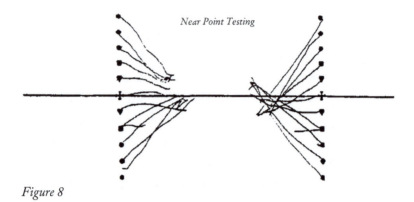

Figure 8

Conclusion

According to my model, a star pattern in which both apices are well formed, but meet below the line, depicts a problem of binocular coordination. This level of dysfunction has a relatively mild effect on the patient's sense of well-being. The pattern is commonly associated with near-point stress.

When the drawings end above the line but fail to meet in a definite apex, there is a more severe spatial organization problem. This pattern signals a temporal–spatial mismatch, and the individual's behavior will indicate a greater degree of stress.

As problems with the "where" system increase in severity, the digressions of pattern execution will increase. The key is that there is a mismatch in the magnitude of frontal plane design between the right and left fields. This represents an individual who has problems organizing the space world, and at the same time is unable to orient self in personal space. It is not uncommon for these people to relate instances of panic behavior.

In the Kaplan Star, I believe we are viewing stereopsis on an unconscious perceptual level. The organization of the patterns is influenced by the time it takes to process perceptions of a global pattern. Interaction of different areas of the brain is required to perform the act of producing the star. Julesz's work cited in Szentágothai and Arbib (1975), on "cyclopean perception," shows that fusion of the two retinal images must precede pattern recognition. Unconscious perception precedes conscious identification. Interference with the process results in disorders of behavior that are reflected in the Star pattern.

In my clinical experience, the Kaplan Star's predictive power equals or even exceeds traditional approaches in terms of identifying behaviors related to visual dysfunction. Using the Kaplan Star allows professionals to diagnose patients' problems with high sensitivity and specificity. The test is both time- and cost-effective and produces few false positives, making it ideal for routine clinical use.

The Kaplan Nonverbal Battery

The tasks in the Kaplan Nonverbal Battery are arranged logically in a hierarchy that allows an observer to see how the child deals with increasing demands on the visual system. The initial tasks focus on visual perception in isolation, while succeeding tasks require the patient to coordinate visual, vestibular, proprioceptive, auditory, and gravitational input.

In each step, the clinician assesses the patient's posture, attention, and disposition in response to a visual demand, both before and after applying ambient prism lenses. To codify the results, I recommend using a score sheet (see the "Perceptual Analysis Score Sheet" sample provided at the end of this appendix).

Pre-Test Evaluation

You will be able to pick up many clues before formal testing begins, simply by observing your patients when they arrive. The vision problems of developmentally disabled children, and autistic children in particular, will manifest themselves in a variety of ways. Many patients will toe-walk, toe in, or touch the walls when they walk. These patients are unable to handle both self and space simultaneously. They will flap their hands to achieve balance, run their hands along the wall for tactile guidance, or toe in for orientation. They will walk on their toes because they do not trust themselves in space, and thus try to hold onto the ground for as long as possible. They often take shorter steps, which is also an attempt to maintain contact with the ground. Rather than sitting smoothly, some will need to feel for the chair and will sit awkwardly.

Your initial observation can also reveal signs of the functional scoliosis that often occurs in response to visual problems. This is important, because this problem can frequently be reversed with therapy

Once your patient is relaxed and ready to participate in testing, you can begin your formal evaluation. Here are the tasks, in order, that make up the Kaplan Nonverbal Battery.

Task 1: video viewing seated

For this task, two chairs are positioned side by side, four or five feet in front of a 19-inch color TV monitor. One chair is for the patient, and the other for the parent or caregiver. The chair height must be low enough to allow the patient to place his or her feet flat on the floor. Parents are asked not to give any directions to the child, such as "sit up straight," because it is important to observe the child's natural head and body posture.

Parents or caregivers are instructed to bring along one of the patient's favorite videos. For the first test, the clinician inserts the video and observes the child's behavior before and after ambient prism lenses are applied. It is important to take very detailed notes, and I also recommend videotaping each session so it will be possible to review the visit later as an observer rather than as a participant. Among the factors to evaluate:

- Does the patient pay attention to the video? Is that attention brief or sustained? Is the patient attending to both visual and auditory input?

- Does the patient tilt his or her head while watching, or watch out of the corner of one eye?

- Does the patient exhibit self-stimulatory behavior such as hand-flapping or tapping while watching the video?

- Is he or she relaxed or tense?

- Does the patient exhibit strabismus/exotropia/esotropia?

Over 20 years, I have seen every possible variation of television watching. Some patients sit up straight while facing the screen. Others sit to the side or tilt their head sideways, avoiding binocular vision because both eyes cannot efficiently fixate on the same point. Some patients sit for only a short time, and then get up to touch the screen or play with the dials. Many engage in repetitive, self-stimulatory behaviors, commonly rocking side-to-side (using gravity to enhance their body awareness) or front-to-back (in an attempt to achieve depth perception). Some wrap their feet around the chair, sit on their hands, or grip the chair arms tightly, signaling that they cannot attend simultaneously to body sense and visual demands.

Often, the type of video the child prefers can be as instructive as the child's behavior. For instance, one of my patients chose to watch a tape of the Miss America pageant over and over, while another preferred tapes of the weather channel and a still another would only watch the credits of shows. Sometimes children will be comfortable watching certain sections of a video, but cover their ears, scream, or turn their eyes away during other sections. Such behaviors provide valuable insights into the type and amount of visual and sensory input a patient is capable of handling.

Once the clinician formulates an accurate idea of the patient's level of performance on this task, it is time to move to the next stage: determining which ambient prism lenses will successfully alter this performance. For this purpose, I use a set of standard optical frames in two sizes (for children and adults), color-coded so that it is easy to identify the types of yoked prisms: base-up, base-down, base-right, or base-left.

Typically, it makes sense to begin with the lenses most likely to precipitate a change that will be observable to the clinician, to the child's parent, and, most importantly, to the child. As each set of ambient prism lenses is applied, the clinician observes for changes in posture, attention, and disposition.

No two children are alike, but most children will clearly signal when a pair of lenses creates a significant change. One of my patients, for example, watched the television while poking one finger up his nostril, higher and higher. When I applied the correct ambient lenses, he removed his finger from his nose. When I gave him a second pair, with prisms in the opposite directions, up went the finger again. Another patient, a large and imposing autistic young man, maintained a constant, rhythmic running of his fingers through his hair, until I found the lenses that relieved his stress. With these lenses in place, he sat calmly and held his hands at rest, quietly watching the video.

Some children will reveal that a particular set of lenses is effective by exhibiting marked changes in attention. One autistic boy, for instance, listened to the sound of the video but turned his head away to avoid watching it. Given the correct pair of ambient prism lenses, he was able to process both visual and auditory input without becoming overwhelmed. In other patients, a response to lenses will be signaled by reductions or escalations in rocking, hair-pulling, groin-touching, leg movement, self-injurious behaviors, vocalizations, laughing, or facial grimacing.

Task 2: video viewing with balance board

Task 1 evaluates vision in relative isolation, requiring only eye movements and not visually guided actions. Task 2 is a greater challenge, because it requires integration of the visual, proprioceptive, and gravitational systems.

This task is performed in the same room used for Task 1. This time, the patient is asked to stand on a balance board (16 inches by 16 inches, with a three-inch by two-inch fulcrum) while watching the same video used in Task 1. The child's responses will tell the clinician, on a "micro" level, how well the child can handle multisensory experiences in everyday life.

Experience has taught me to modify this procedure when a patient displays severe problems in orientation. For instance, if the child is so disoriented that the caregiver needs to hold his or her hand until the lenses are in place, I will begin with the patient seated on the balance board. Once the patient gains confidence, we can then switch to the standing position.

Again, the patient's reactions are tested both with and without ambient prism lenses. The clinician looks for changes in posture, attention, and disposition, as well as assessing the child's level of performance—can the child successfully balance while watching the video? How skillfully? For how long?—during the no-lenses and lenses conditions. When the right lenses are applied, the change between the no-lens and lens conditions should be readily detectable.

Task 3: ball play

This task again ups the ante, by requiring a patient to exhibit visual motor coordination, visual spatial judgment (timing), and intersensory coordination of localization. To catch a ball successfully, an individual must correlate the internal model of time and the external model of space. Any difficulty in making this temporal–spatial match will result in poor performance, a feeling of apprehension, and eventually a reduction in attention as the individual becomes frustrated by continual failure.

For this activity the clinician will need a plastic baseball tethered to a string and set at chest level. When body schema is a severe problem, the patient can initially perform this task while seated, reducing the need for intersensory coordination. If a patient's deficits are so severe that catching the ball is impossible, switching from a ball to a balloon will slow the speed and allow the patient more time.

During this task the clinician notes how well the patient attends to the ball, whether the individual moves toward the ball or attempts to dodge it, and whether the individual catches the ball itself or the string—all clues that can point to specific visual deficits. For example, one ten-year-old autistic girl who held her head constantly tilted displayed a "flight reaction" when the ball on the string was thrown in her direction. When I placed the correct ambient lenses on her, she stood her ground and reached out to catch the ball. The diagnosis: convergence insufficiency, a mismatch between where she perceived objects and where they actually existed. Her problem was a severe deficit in spatial perception, and her solution, in order to survive, was avoidance.

Once a clinician has a good idea of the patient's level of performance in this task, the task is repeated with the lenses that proved most beneficial during the earlier tasks. In most cases, patients will experience an immediate and dramatic improvement in performance. (This change is so marked that one response I frequently hear from verbal patients is, "What happened—did you throw the ball slower?") In addition to confirming the correct selection of ambient prism lenses, this change will motivate the patient to continue with testing and vision therapy.

The ball task also provides an excellent opportunity to give parents some first-hand insight into how disabling their children's visual deficits are, and how beneficial vision therapy can be. As parents observe the changes in their children, they typically ask, "What are these lenses? How do they work?" I find it easier to show them than to tell them.

Most of the parents of my patients have mild or moderate visual impairments themselves, but aren't aware of these problems. Often, when I throw a ball toward them, they exhibit some version of the symptoms their child has displayed. They quickly apologize, saying, "I haven't played in a long time," or, "I never really played ball." However, when I place the correct ambient prism lenses on the parents, and their ability immediately improves, they become quite excited. Like their children, they do not consciously feel the changes in their visual–motor behavior, but they can easily tell that the glasses are causing a significant difference.

Sometimes, however, the parents are experts at ball catching, without the help of ambient prism lenses. In these cases, I take a different tack. "In your child's case," I tell them, "I made them better; however, in your case, I will cause you to perform poorly." The next time I throw the ball, I have the parents wear disruptive ambient prisms, which precipitate a time–space mismatch of eyes and hands. Immediately they become tense and grow irritated by the difficulty in succeeding at a formerly simple task—and they better understand just how unfriendly the world can seem to a child with severe visual dysfunction.

Task 4: seated pursuits and Task 5: standing pursuits

For the first of these tasks the patient is seated in a comfortable position with the feet touching the floor. The examiner is seated directly in front of the patient. The target can be a Bruce wand (a rod with a metal ball on the end), a shiny ball, or a finger, but I use a puppet figure placed on the head of a lit flashlight. This catches the attention of pediatric patients, and also amuses and relaxes adults.

The clinician first asks the patient to keep his or her eyes on the lit puppet, which is moved in a circular pattern followed by direct movements through the cardinal meridian. The clinician watches for the following:

- Can the patient sustain eye movement?

- Are the movements jumpy (saccadic)?

- Does the child follow with eyes alone, eyes and head, or even the body?

- Does the child reach with a hand to grab the object, or direct the eyes by pointing?

When there is a total lack of eye movement, the clinician should change the target to a bell. This will show the examiner if auditory input can influence eye movement and, if so, to what extent. If neither the lit puppet nor the bell elicits movement, the clinician should ask the patient to point at the puppet. Often, the addition of proprioceptive feedback will cue eye movement.

The clinician then repeats the pursuit procedure, this time with the patient standing. Perceptual style and degree of eye movement dysfunction will dictate whether a child performs better while sitting or while standing. In either condition, the clinician watches to see if the child holds his or her breath, becomes hyperactive, or totally avoids the stimulus. These behaviors raise concerns about the visual stability centers, which receive information regarding the motor outflow to the eye muscle (the third, fourth and sixth cranial nerves). The ability to judge observed movements depends on the interplay of information from these centers, which are responsible for the voluntary control of eye movements.

In both conditions, seated and standing, the testing is repeated with ambient prism lenses. The response of a child in these conditions is very significant for prognosis. For example, if I can solicit improved eye movement with ambient prisms during this task while testing a nonverbal or verbally delayed child with pervasive developmental disorder, I can in good conscience tell the parents that in four to six months we will get language.

Task 6: mirror balance on one foot

In this task the patient is asked to balance on one foot in front of a mirror. This tests a patient's ability to coordinate sensory modalities, as well as providing the clinician with a clearer picture of the child's developmental level. By the age of five, according to the Gesell Battery of Child Development, children should be able to sustain balance on one foot for the count of ten while looking at themselves in a mirror. Those who cannot may have significant issues with body schema.

Some patients have significant problems in orienting themselves during this task because they cannot coordinate visual and vestibular input. These patients may have problems such as vertigo, motion sickness, and fear of heights.

Over time, the clinician will discover that some children place great importance on viewing themselves in a mirror, while others avoid their reflected image at all costs. This is a matter of perceptual style, and will be highly relevant later in designing a therapy program.

This task is performed with the patient standing first on the right foot, and then on the left (or vice versa). In each of these conditions, the task is performed first without and then with the ambient prism lenses. In each instance the clinician observes posture, attention, and disposition, and notes the patient's ability to sustain the posture, the amount of tilt, the position of hands and arms, and where visual attention is directed.

Task 7: video balance on one foot

This task is similar to the previous one (mirror balance on one foot) except that the patient is asked to balance while watching a video on television. The results of this and the mirror task offer the clinician insight into whether the patient is field dependent (attends to space) or field independent (attends to self). This information can be used later to design an effective visual management program.

Task 8: balloon play

This procedure is performed standing, and requires a ten-inch balloon. The clinician demonstrates to the child how to hit the balloon up in the air, first with one hand and then with the other, while counting from one to ten. The activity is then repeated, this time using the ambient prism lenses that have proven most effective.

In this task, the patient's visual system is forced to interact with both general and specific motor skills. To succeed at the task, a patient must be able to use the hands alternately, track the balloon when it goes over his or her head, and maintain a limited range of body movement. Poor performers tend to lose the balloon when it goes over their heads, or have trouble hitting it accurately enough to make it rise above eye level. In addition, they often must move excessively to keep up with the balloon, because they tend to hit it sideways rather than up.

Task 9: walk and sit

This task requires two chairs, placed eight to ten feet apart. The clinician asks the child to walk from one chair to the other and then sit down without touching the chair with his or her hands. The task is then repeated with the child wearing disruptive yoked prisms, using a magnitude of 15–20 diopters. With base-down lenses, the child will typically knock over the chair. In the base-up condition, the child will come up short of the chair. With base-right prisms, the child will sit left of the chair, and with base-left, to the right of the chair.

The use of disruptive lenses allows the clinician to discover how a patient reacts to having his or her world visually transformed in a dramatic way. Does the individual walk slowly, or rush? Does he or she go down on all fours, and crawl across the floor? Does the patient shuffle cautiously, or lift the feet? Does the patient show fear and rip off the glasses, or seem delighted by the reactivation of previously "turned off" visual processes in order to understand this new visual world? All of these reactions will tell the clinician how to proceed when planning a visual management program.

A note about handling tactile defensiveness

As you conduct the tests I've outlined, one problem you are likely to encounter in patients with learning differences, autism, or related problems is "tactile defensiveness"—an extreme sensitivity to touch, which can cause a patient to cry, withdraw, or even strike out when touched. Frequently, patients with tactile defensiveness will exhibit associated symptoms such as hyperactivity and distractability. Patients who are tactilely defensive frequently resist wearing prism lenses, even when they discover that the glasses help them to see and perform better.

In working with patients who react strongly to tactile stimuli, it is important to understand the causes of their problem—and one of these causes is poor visual processing. Over many centuries we've evolved to depend increasingly on higher-level visual and auditory senses, which allow us to quickly inhibit and modulate our actions and emotional responses to stimuli. Many children with autism or related disabilities, however, are locked into trusting touch, taste, and smell for movement arousal for fight or flight. Lacking an accurate body schema, and dependent on lower-level sensory input to identify threats, they survive by overreacting to stimuli that the rest of us can accurately and quickly dismiss with the aid of efficient visual processes.

When a patient displays tactile defensiveness, and associated hyperactivity and distractability, a struggle over wearing the prism lenses is likely to occur. Red flags include head tilting, visual avoidance, hyperactive movements, and emotional outbursts in response to tasks. To make it easier for tactilely defensive patients to accept wearing glasses, I introduce the glasses in an environment in which the field of view allows for the least possible amount of eye movement (for instance, while the patient is seated and watching television). In my experience, 80 percent of patients will accept the lenses immediately under these conditions, while the other 20 percent will accept them more gradually. To a great degree, a patient's ability to accept the glasses varies according to age, intelligence, and efficiency of auditory processing. The important thing is to persist, even in the face of strong initial resistance, if you are confident that the glasses will help your patient.

Perceptual Analysis Score Sheet

Patient's name:_____

Date:_____ Age:_____

HAB = baseline performance (using lenses if patient has a previous prescription)
BU = base-up lenses
BD = base-down lenses
BR = base-right lenses
BL = base-left lenses

1. VIDEO VIEWING SEATED				
	HEAD POSTURE	**BODY POSTURE**	**VISUAL ATTENTION**	**DISPOSITION**
HAB	4 3 2 1 0	4 3 2 1 0	4 3 2 1 0	4 3 2 1 0
BU ( )	4 3 2 1 0	4 3 2 1 0	4 3 2 1 0	4 3 2 1 0
BD ( )	4 3 2 1 0	4 3 2 1 0	4 3 2 1 0	4 3 2 1 0
BR	4 3 2 1 0	4 3 2 1 0	4 3 2 1 0	4 3 2 1 0
BL	4 3 2 1 0	4 3 2 1 0	4 3 2 1 0	4 3 2 1 0

2. VIDEO VIEWING WITH BALANCE BOARD				
	HEAD POSTURE	**BODY POSTURE**	**VISUAL ATTENTION**	**DISPOSITION**
HAB	4 3 2 1 0	4 3 2 1 0	4 3 2 1 0	4 3 2 1 0
BU ( )	4 3 2 1 0	4 3 2 1 0	4 3 2 1 0	4 3 2 1 0
BD ( )	4 3 2 1 0	4 3 2 1 0	4 3 2 1 0	4 3 2 1 0

3. BALL PLAY			
	MOVEMENT/ POSTURE	ATTENTION	DISPOSITION
HAB	4 3 2 1 0	4 3 2 1 0	4 3 2 1 0
( )	4 3 2 1 0	4 3 2 1 0	4 3 2 1 0

4. SEATED PURSUITS			
	MOVEMENT/ POSTURE	ATTENTION	DISPOSITION
HAB	4 3 2 1 0	4 3 2 1 0	4 3 2 1 0
( )	4 3 2 1 0	4 3 2 1 0	4 3 2 1 0

5. STANDING PURSUITS			
	MOVEMENT/ POSTURE	ATTENTION	DISPOSITION
HAB	4 3 2 1 0	4 3 2 1 0	4 3 2 1 0
( )	4 3 2 1 0	4 3 2 1 0	4 3 2 1 0

6. MIRROR BALANCE ON ONE FOOT				
	HEAD POSTURE	BODY POSTURE	VISUAL ATTENTION	DISPOSITION
HAB	4 3 2 1 0	4 3 2 1 0	4 3 2 1 0	4 3 2 1 0
HAB R	4 3 2 1 0	4 3 2 1 0	4 3 2 1 0	4 3 2 1 0
HAB L	4 3 2 1 0	4 3 2 1 0	4 3 2 1 0	4 3 2 1 0
( )	4 3 2 1 0	4 3 2 1 0	4 3 2 1 0	4 3 2 1 0
( )	4 3 2 1 0	4 3 2 1 0	4 3 2 1 0	4 3 2 1 0

7. VIDEO BALANCE ON ONE FOOT				
	HEAD POSTURE	**BODY POSTURE**	**VISUAL ATTENTION**	**DISPOSITION**
HAB R	4 3 2 1 0	4 3 2 1 0	4 3 2 1 0	4 3 2 1 0
HAB L	4 3 2 1 0	4 3 2 1 0	4 3 2 1 0	4 3 2 1 0
( )	4 3 2 1 0	4 3 2 1 0	4 3 2 1 0	4 3 2 1 0
( )	4 3 2 1 0	4 3 2 1 0	4 3 2 1 0	4 3 2 1 0

8. BALLOON PLAY			
	MOVEMENT	**ATTENTION**	**DISPOSITION**
HAB	4 3 2 1 0	4 3 2 1 0	4 3 2 1 0
( )	4 3 2 1 0	4 3 2 1 0	4 3 2 1 0
( )	4 3 2 1 0	4 3 2 1 0	4 3 2 1 0

9. WALK AND SIT			
	MOVEMENT/ POSTURE	**ATTENTION**	**DISPOSITION**
HAB R	4 3 2 1 0	4 3 2 1 0	4 3 2 1 0
HAB L	4 3 2 1 0	4 3 2 1 0	4 3 2 1 0
( )	4 3 2 1 0	4 3 2 1 0	4 3 2 1 0
( )	4 3 2 1 0	4 3 2 1 0	4 3 2 1 0

References

Atkinson, R.C. and Shiffrin R.M. (1968) "Human Memory: A Proposed System and its Control Processes." In K.W. Spence and J.T. Spence *The Psychology of Learning and Motivation (Volume 2)*. New York: Academic Press, 89–195.

Bridgeman, B. (1992) "On the evolution of consciousness and language." *Psycoloquy 3*, 15.

Byrd, J.A. III (1988) "Current theories on the etiology of idiopathic scoliosis." *Clinical Orthopaedics and Related Research 229*, 114–119.

Dolezal, H. (1982) *Living in a World Transformed*. New York: Academic Press.

Dunn, R. and Griggs, S.A. (2000) *Practical Approaches to Using Learning Styles in Higher Education*. Westport, CT: Praeger.

Flach, F. (1990) *Rickie*. New York: Fawcett Columbine.

Flach, F. and Kaplan, M. (1983) "Visual perceptual dysfunction in psychiatric patients." *Comprehensive Psychiatry 24*, 4, 304–311.

Flach, F., Kaplan, M., Bengelsdorf, H., Orlowski, B., Friedenthal, S., Weisbard, J., and Carmody, D. (1992) "Visual perceptual dysfunction: schizophrenic and affective disorders vs. controls." *Journal of Neuropsychiatry and Clinical Neurosciences 4*, 422–427.

Gesell, A. (1950) *Vision: Its Development in Infant and Child*. London: H. Hamilton.

Herman, R., Mixon, J., Fisher, A., Maulucci, R. and Stuyck, J. (1985) "Idiopathic Scoliosis and the Central Nervous System: A Motor Control Problem: The Harrington Lecture, 1983, Scoliosis Research Society." *Spine 10*, 1, 1–14.

Kaplan, M. (1975) "An optometric approach to motion sickness." *Optical Journal and Review of Optometry 112*, 9.

Kaplan, M., Carmody, D.P. and Gaydos, A. (1996) "Postural orientation modifications in autism in response to ambient lenses." *Child Psychiatry and Human Development 27*, 2, 81–91.

Kaplan, M., Edelson, S.M. and Seip, J.L. (1998) "Behavioral changes in autistic individuals as a result of wearing ambient transitional prism lenses." *Child Psychiatry & Human Development 29*, 1, 65–76.

Kaplan, M., Rimland, B. and Edelson, S.M. (1999) "Strabismus in autism spectrum disorder." *Focus on Autism and Other Developmental Disabilities 14*, 2, 101–105.

Kolb, D.A. (1984) *Experiential Learning: Experience as the Source of Learning and Development (Volume 1)*. Englewood Cliffs, NJ: Prentice-Hall.

LeDoux, J. (1998) *The Emotional Brain: The Mysterious Underpinnings of Emotional Life*. New York: Simon & Schuster.

Oman, C.M. (1990) "Motion sickness: A synthesis and evaluation of the sensory conflict theory." *Canadian Journal of Physiology and Pharmacology 68*, 2, 294–303.

Ratey, J. (2002) *A User's Guide to the Brain: Perception, Attention, and the Four Theaters of the Brain.* New York: Vintage.

Selye, H. (1995) *Stress Without Distress.* New York: Signet.

Sokhadze, G., Kaplan, M., Sokhadze, E.M., Edelson, S.M. et al. (2012) "Effects of ambient prism lenses on autonomic reactivity to emotional stimuli in autism." Presentation to the International Meeting for Autism Research (IMFAR), Toronto, May 18.

Szentagothai, J. and Arbib, M. (1975) *Conceptual Models of Neural Organization.* Cambridge, MA: MIT Press.

Index